SCIENTIFIC INQUIRY IN NURSING EDUCATION

ADVANCING THE SCIENCE

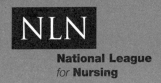

National League
for **Nursing**

SCIENTIFIC INQUIRY IN NURSING EDUCATION

ADVANCING THE SCIENCE

Edited by:

Barbara J. Patterson, PhD, RN, ANEF

Anne M. Krouse, PhD, MBA, RN-BC

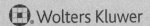. Wolters Kluwer

Philadelphia • Baltimore • New York • London
Buenos Aires • Hong Kong • Sydney • Tokyo

Acquisitions Editor: Sherry Dickinson
Product Development Editor: Dan Reilly
Production Project Manager: Priscilla Crater
Design Coordinator: Terry Mallon
Illustration Coordinator: Jennifer Clements
Manufacturing Coordinator: Karin Duffield
Marketing Manager: Todd McQueston
Prepress Vendor: Aptara, Inc.

Copyright © 2017 National League for Nursing

Patterson B.J., and Krouse, A.M. (2017). *Scientific Inquiry in Nursing Education: Advancing the Science.* Washington, DC: National League for Nursing.

9 8 7 6 5 4 3 2 1

Printed in the United States of America

Library of Congress Cataloging-in-Publication Data

Names: Patterson, Barbara J., editor. | Krouse, Anne M., editor. | National
    League for Nursing, issuing body.
Title: Scientific inquiry in nursing education : advancing the science /
    edited by Barbara J. Patterson, Anne M. Krouse.
Description: [Washington, DC] : National League for Nursing ; Philadelphia :
    Wolters Kluwer, [2017] | Includes bibliographical references.
Identifiers: LCCN 2016028191 | ISBN 9781934758281 (alk. paper)
Subjects: | MESH: Nursing Education Research | Evidence-Based Nursing |
    Nursing Theory
Classification: LCC RT81.5 | NLM WY 18 | DDC 610.73072–dc23
LC record available at https://lccn.loc.gov/2016028191

DRC0916

About the Editors

Barbara J. Patterson, PhD, RN, ANEF is a distinguished professor and director of the doctoral program in the School of Nursing, associate dean for scholarship and inquiry, and chair of the Institutional Review Board at Widener University in Chester, Pennsylvania. She received a diploma in nursing from Millard Fillmore Hospital School of Nursing, bachelor of science in nursing from D'Youville College, master of science in nursing from the University of Southern Maine, and a doctoral degree from the University of Rhode Island. She has teaching experience with prelicensure nursing students in advanced medical-surgical nursing, gerontology, and research and with doctoral students in qualitative research, nursing science and theory, lead-

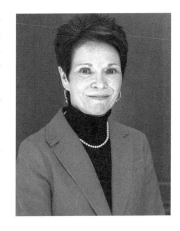

ership, and dissertation advisement. She has chaired more than 40 doctoral dissertations, many of which investigated nursing education topics. Dr. Patterson has presented and published extensively in nursing education. Her research and publications are in the areas of social support and aging, evidence-based teaching, veterans care, and leadership in nursing education. She is faculty for the Nurse Faculty Leadership Academy of Sigma Theta Tau International, where she works with novice nurse educators and individual leadership development. Dr. Patterson was chair of the Research Review Panel for the National League for Nursing (NLN) from 2012 to 2015, which reviews research grants for nursing education. She has been active on several task groups at the NLN, specific to educational preparation of nurse educators and nursing education research priorities. Dr. Patterson is also the Research Briefs editor for *Nursing Education Perspectives*.

Anne M. Krouse, PhD, MBA, RN-BC is a professor in the School of Nursing at Widener University in Chester, Pennsylvania, where she also holds the position of associate provost for learning spaces and strategic initiatives. Dr. Krouse is also the coordinator of the Executive Nurse Leadership program. Her teaching experience is in the areas of maternal-child health, nursing education, leadership, informatics, and health policy. She was awarded the Fitz Dixon Innovation in Teaching Award in 2012 for her work in teaching health policy. Her research and publications primarily have been in the areas of nursing education, leadership, and maternal-child health. Dr. Krouse is a member of the National League for Nursing Public Policy Committee.

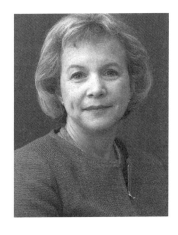

About the Contributors

Lisa Day, PhD, RN, CNE is an associate clinical professor at Duke University School of Nursing in Durham, North Carolina, and has consulted on many nursing education–related projects, including the first phase of the Carnegie Foundation National Nursing Education Study, a project funded by the Robert Wood Johnson Foundation. She is a coauthor of the landmark publication *Educating Nurses: A Call for Radical Transformation* reporting the results of the Carnegie study and has provided faculty development workshops for schools of nursing in the United States and Canada. She is certified as a nurse educator by the National League for Nursing and was one of five faculty members from schools of nursing and medicine in the United States selected to participate in the Josiah Macy Jr. Foundation Faculty Scholar Program, 2013–2015. Dr. Day is working on a pilot study to test the feasibility of a learning innovation for CNA, LPN, and RN education.

Barbara Manz Friesth, PhD, RN is a faculty member in the Department of Community and Health Systems at Indiana University School of Nursing (IUSON). She is also the assistant dean of learning resources and the codirector of the Encouraging Learning, Innovation, and Technology Excellence (ELITE) Center. In her administrative roles, she is responsible for providing leadership and vision for integration of instructional technologies into curricula of the IUSON programs, including online and distance accessible learning. Dr. Friesth has served as a coinvestigator or consultant on several grants and projects related to distance education in nursing programs.

Lynne Porter Lewallen, PhD, RN, CNE, ANEF is a professor and assistant dean for academic affairs at the University of North Carolina at Greensboro School of Nursing. She is an accreditation site visitor and team chair and has experience speaking and consulting about program evaluation and nursing education research. Her research interests include health promotion in pregnancy and prenatal care and clinical evaluation in nursing education. She is active with the National League for Nursing, serving on the Research Review Panel and the Editorial Board of *Nursing Education Perspectives*.

Bette Mariani, PhD, RN is an assistant professor of nursing at Villanova University College of Nursing. Her expertise and research is in the area of simulation development, research instrument development, and debriefing in all types of simulations. Her research is focused on exploring the outcomes of simulation as a teaching-learning strategy with standardized patients with disabilities, as well as in the area of medication and patient safety. Dr. Mariani's research also focuses on instrument development and psychometric testing for simulation. She is cochair of the International Nursing Association for Clinical Simulation and Learning (INACSL) Research Committee and contributed to the INACSL Standards on Simulation Design. She has published and presented in the area of simulation, leadership development through simulation, and instrument development and psychometric testing.

Karen H. Morin, PhD, RN, FAAN, ANEF is a professor emerita of the University of Wisconsin at Milwaukee. She has extensive experience in nursing education and expertise in doctoral education (PhD and DNP), leadership, curriculum development, and program evaluation. She received the Excellence in Teaching Award from the National League for Nursing in 2003 and the Excellence in Nursing Education Award from the Association of Women's Health, Obstetric, and Neonatal Nurses in 1999. Dr. Morin also is the director of the Center for Nursing Inquiry at Bronson Methodist Hospital in Kalamazoo, Michigan, where she assists staff nurses with the development and implementation of quality improvement projects and research. She also serves as an associate editor for the *Journal of Nursing Education*.

Teresa Shellenbarger, PhD, RN, CNE, ANEF is a professor in the Department of Nursing and Allied Health Professions at Indiana University of Pennsylvania in Indiana, Pennsylvania. She has been a nurse educator for more than 25 years and has taught in multiple levels of nursing education. An accomplished author, researcher, and nursing leader, Dr. Shellenbarger has expertise in program development, assessment and evaluation, nursing education research, and faculty role development. She is a National League for Nursing (NLN) certified nurse educator and was inducted as an inaugural fellow in the NLN Academy of Nursing Education.

Darrell Spurlock, Jr., PhD, RN, NEA-BC, ANEF is a nursing education researcher and Associate Professor of Nursing at Widener University in Chester, PA. With an academic background in both psychology and nursing, Dr. Spurlock's research on high-stakes testing in nursing education is widely quoted in scholarly papers and textbooks, cited in regulatory and legal opinions and guidelines, and has stimulated numerous lines of inquiry by other nursing education researchers. Dr. Spurlock's primary interest is in building the science of nursing education through original research, instrument development, and promotion of evidence-based nursing education practices.

Foreword

I began teaching in the early 1970s. It was clear to me as a young educator that we did not have all the answers for how to best teach our students. I was frustrated by the extensive use of the written nursing care plan as the only means to teach clinical reasoning. I saw little relationship between what students wrote in the 2 a.m.–produced care plan and what the plan actually did for the patient the following day. It gave me little insight into how students actually thought about evolving clinical situations and gave me little guidance in how to coach them. I was doing what most young educators do—I taught as I was taught. But my frustrations led me back to school—this time in an educational psychology program, thinking that I might find new ways to help students learn how to think. I was lucky in choosing a program that would give me a good foundation in educational research and in theories that would be useful for guiding my research interests.

When I completed my PhD, I felt well prepared, having completed a rigorous program of study, steeped in cognitive science theories and educational research methods that would advance my program of research in clinical reasoning. I was ready to launch a research career. However, within a few years, the discipline turned its collective energy toward developing our clinical science, focused on patient care issues and concerns, and discouraging efforts in nursing education research. I made a few feeble efforts to shift my focus to clinical science, but my real passion and expertise lay in nursing education research. So I persisted in developing a program of research on clinical judgment that spanned over three decades of work.

I remember one of the arguments of the day: nursing education research could and should be done by educational researchers. Developing the science of learning and translating this science into educational interventions did not require nursing discipline-specific expertise. Despite this prevalent belief, institutional policies that often did not reward educational scholarship, and lack of funding for its support, scores of nursing education researchers persisted in developing a science for nursing education. The National League for Nursing (NLN) has been a stalwart proponent for nursing education scholarship, supporting the nascent Society for Research in Nursing Education in the mid-1980s and providing small grant funds and a frequently updated list of research priorities. The arguments against nursing investment in educational research have been laid to rest. As the Institute of Medicine (IOM) (2011) notes:

> At no time in recent history has there been a greater need for research on nursing education. As health care reform progresses, basic and advanced nursing practices are being defined by the new competencies, yet virtually no evidence exists to support teaching approaches used in nursing education. Additionally, little research has focused on clinical education models or clinical experiences that can help student achieve these competencies even though clinical education constitutes the largest portion of nurses' education costs. (p. 198)

The research priorities identified by both the NLN and the IOM clearly point to the need for discipline-specific research, not simply the application of general learning science to the education of nursing students. For example, both the IOM and NLN place high priority on the "development and testing of instruments to measure learning outcomes" (National League for Nursing, 2016) and "identification or development of an assessment tool to ensure that nurses have acquired the full range of competence required to practice nursing." Developing research-based pedagogies for teaching specific aspects of nursing practice clearly requires discipline-specific knowledge. Although there is a fairly robust body of knowledge related to clinical reasoning in nursing, as the NLN (2016) points out, much work is needed in "identification of innovative approaches to learning that improve clinical reasoning and judgment applied to patient care" (p. 3).

This textbook comes at an ideal time in our development. Each of the topics explored in each of the chapters could take up a full text, and some have. But the contributors have carefully selected content particularly relevant to the beginning researcher in nursing education. This text will be the gateway for the next generation of nursing education scientists.

Christine A. Tanner, PhD, RN
Professor Emerita
Oregon Health and Science University
School of Nursing

Preface

Stevens and Cassidy (1999), almost two decades ago, defined *evidence-based teaching* as "the conscientious, explicit, and judicious use of current best evidence in making decisions about the education of professional nurses" (p. 3). This book focuses on the crucial components of generating the best evidence through empirical inquiry. There has been tremendous growth in the body of research evidence in some areas of teaching and learning in nursing, whereas in other areas the evidence remains limited. It is important to note that this emphasis on research evidence in no way discounts other sources of evidence, such as faculty anecdotal accounts of their teaching practice. The intent of this book is not to elaborate, dispute, or challenge what constitutes the scholarship of teaching and learning or what is meant by scholarly teaching but rather to focus on one aspect—the generation, dissemination, and translation of robust-quality research evidence for implementation in teaching practice.

The increasingly complex and continually evolving health care environment coupled with the growth in the science of learning requires nurse faculty to rethink how they are teaching. How we teach and what we teach is being questioned by multiple stakeholders in higher education, including the public at large. Given these forces, a major impetus for this book was a concern for the quality of the scholarship and research evidence being generated on which nursing faculty were basing their teaching practices. Through multiple dialogues with the book contributors and other colleagues, in addition to the review of research proposals, grants, and publications over many years, the need to strengthen the research being conducted seemed critical.

Research is nursing education is challenging but also rewarding. Triggered through our work with PhD students for more than a decade, we recognized that our students were knowledgeable about the role of the nurse educator, had a strong nursing science foundation, acquired knowledge about teaching and learning theories, and were prepared to conduct research. It was the merging of these areas into a robust meaningful research proposal that was the challenge for us as their doctoral faculty. Many of our students conduct pedagogical research for their dissertations. Guiding them in designing theoretically based, quality studies that would have an impact on nursing education and the science was the goal.

This book hopes to fill a gap in the area of nursing research. It offers a perspective that focuses scientific inquiry directly on our teaching practice. The audience for this book is those scholars interested in conducting and using pedagogical research. There are multiple audiences for this work. Doctoral students, both PhD and DNP, will find the information instrumental in their research, as there is a need to both generate and translate and implement the research. Additionally, novice, experienced, and seasoned nurse faculty who want to conduct research in nursing education, whether at the beginning of their academic careers or at a transition point in their research trajectory, will benefit from the guidance provided in these chapters.

Nurse scientists hold roles and function in a wide variety of contexts, including health care, higher education, or proprietary or community-based organizations. The mission for all nurses is improving the health of the nation and the world. As a practice discipline, we need a culture that supports a community of inquiry—a culture of academics and clinicians working respectfully together through collaborative efforts to move beyond the silos of clinical versus pedagogical research. Quality research is quality research, no matter the context. Faculty teaching practice informs the clinical practice of the students we prepare. Nurse scholars need to be designing and conducting research that connects how students learn, how faculty teach, and patient care outcomes. Clinical and academic nurse scientists, working collaboratively, are in the optimal position to generate this body of knowledge. As a leader in nursing education, the National League for Nursing (NLN) has recognized the importance of this focus in its *Research Priorities in Nursing Education* report (National League for Nursing [NLN], 2016). The research priorities were designed to intentionally link nursing education and practice through the incorporation of the key themes from the National Institute of Nursing Research (NINR) strategic plan to advance the science of health (National Institute of Nursing Research, 2016).

This book is not a traditional book on research methodologies. Many books on research design and statistics exist. The focus of this book is on those elements crucial to designing quality pedagogical studies that support or challenge our current teaching practices, providing methodological support for the 2016–2019 NLN first research priority: "Build the science of nursing education through the discovery and translation of innovative evidence-based strategies" (NLN, 2016, p. 2). The authors who contributed to this book are passionate about research in nursing education and have shared their knowledge and visions for advancement of the science of nursing education through their areas of expertise.

Defining research in nursing education to build a science is the focus of Chapter 1 of the book. It includes a discussion of why it is important to study how we teach and whom we teach, in addition to the impact of these findings. As research scientists, nurse faculty conceptualize, design, and disseminate empirical studies to provide knowledge to support the teaching and learning of students. The evidence that is generated is the foundation for teaching practice.

The connection between theory and research is often a challenging one for nurse scientists. Chapter 2 examines the possibilities for theory use in research in nursing education. Theory is the adhesive that logically joins all of the pieces of a research study together. Whether theory informs the research question or provides structure for an intervention, the role of theory to advance knowledge is foundational.

Finding a focus as to where to start a research study is often the challenge for research scientists. Although there are many potential areas for investigation that contribute to the science, the impact of a focused program of research is greater. Chapter 3 guides researchers from finding a topic to identifying outcome measures. Searching for funding sources and writing the grant proposal can be an intimidating but necessary task if we seek to advance the science beyond single-site descriptive studies. Grant preparation strategies are explored in this chapter.

Measurement of constructs in nursing education is a fundamental requirement for knowledge development. The constructs that are often measured in education include knowledge, attitudes, beliefs, and abilities. Addressing the NLN (2016) call for the "development and testing of instruments for nursing education research to measure learning outcomes and linkages to patient care" (p. 2), Chapter 4 includes practical guidance in the rigorous measurement of education concepts in nursing education. There is a discussion of measurement theory, principles for selecting measures, the process of instrument development, and some key considerations in the development of a robust scientific inquiry.

The importance of design in the development of educational intervention is the focus of Chapter 5. Theory is critical to the design of interventions, as it provides the framework for replication of studies and the advancement of knowledge. Design-based educational research recognizes the contextual variables that may affect the outcomes of an intervention. Refinement of interventions through empirical testing can provide the evidence to support best practices for teaching and learning, which speaks directly to the NLN (2016) call for the "translation of research outcomes into evidence-informed educational practices" (p. 2).

Chapter 6 focuses on the ethical conduct of research in the educational setting. There is a discussion of the challenges and key issues to consider when applying the principles of respect, beneficence, and justice in conducting research with students. Although students may be the best to inform the teaching-learning process, they may be vulnerable when used as research participants. With an increasing concern for scientific misconduct and research integrity, nurse scientists must be cognizant of best practices in human subjects research conducted in the educational context.

The data are collected, and the steps of analyzing and interpreting the data are the next challenge. Implementing best practices to manage, analyze, and interpret data are highlighted in Chapter 7. To address relevant research questions in nursing education, investigators must be knowledgeable of the potential pitfalls and issues that may surface in this phase of a research project. What constitutes the data and the strategies to manage the data need to be considered prior to collection of the data. With quantitative analysis, inviting a statistician to join the research team can provide valuable input to enhance the knowledge contribution. These considerations are critical to building the science of nursing education, as emphasized by the NLN (2016) call for the "creation of robust multi-site, multi-method research designs that address critical education issues" (p. 2). In addition, there is a discussion of Big Data and its role in generating knowledge.

Dissemination of the evidence is the emphasis of Chapter 8. To change educational culture, the processes of presenting and publishing are critical. There is consideration of the importance of translating and integrating empirical evidence into one's teaching practice and the challenges that may be encountered. Steps to promote this phase of the research process within an educational context are offered. As the body of evidence in nursing education grows, there is a need for more integrative and systematic reviews, meta-analysis and metasynthesis studies as noted in the NLN (2016) call for "meta-analysis and meta-synthesis informing the state of the science" (p. 2). The advancement of knowledge in nursing education and educational policy development depends on these next steps.

The last two chapters of the book include presentations of the challenges and key issues in conducting and generating evidence in simulation (Chapter 9) and distance education (Chapter 10). Chapter 9 highlights the research priorities for simulation available from national organizations to guide investigators in moving the science of simulation practice forward. The foundation for a robust simulation study hinges on engaging and collaborating with stakeholders, a theoretical framework, and a strategic plan. Educational outcomes depend on the rigor that is employed in all phases of the study. Chapter 10 focuses on the need for common language and definitions in research on distance education to generate a sound body of evidence to support teaching practices. Methodological considerations in the conduct of research in this area include the use of a theoretical framework to guide the study, the need for a robust multisite study design, and the consideration of research priorities that will advance the science.

This book fills a void in the area of nursing education and research books. It addresses the need for rigorous study designs that are theoretically based using reliable and valid measures that will move the discipline forward. The book is designed for those who want to be at the forefront of research in nursing education to advance the science to effectively teach and prepare nursing students as competent practitioners, no matter the level of their education.

Barbara J. Patterson, PhD, RN, ANEF
Anne M. Krouse, PhD, MBA, RN-BC

References

National Institute of Nursing Research. (2016). *Implementing NINR's strategic plan: Key themes.* Retrieved June 10, 2016, from http://www.ninr.nih.gov/aboutninr/keythemes

National League for Nursing. (2016). *NLN research priorities in nursing education.* Retrieved June 10, 2016, from http://www.nln.org/professional-development-programs/research/research-priorities-in-nursing-education

Stevens, K. R., & Cassidy, V. R. (1999). *Evidence-based teaching: Current research in nursing education.* Boston: Jones & Bartlett.

Acknowledgments

Without the intellectual stimulation, support, and encouragement from the NLN staff, our colleagues, and students, this book would not have been possible. You have our thanks and gratitude.

Barbara J. Patterson & Anne M. Krouse
April 2016

Contents

About the Editors   v

About the Contributors   vi

Foreword   viii

Preface   x

Acknowledgments   xiv

List of Figures and Tables   xvi

CHAPTER 1   **Researching Nursing Education   1**
Barbara J. Patterson, PhD, RN, ANEF and
Anne M. Krouse, PhD, MBA, RN-BC

CHAPTER 2   **The Role of Theory in Nursing Education Research   13**
Lisa Day, PhD, RN, CNE

CHAPTER 3   **Generating the Research Evidence   25**
Lynne Porter Lewallen, PhD, RN, CNE, ANEF

CHAPTER 4   **Measuring Educational Concepts   39**
Darrell Spurlock, Jr., PhD, RN, NEA-BC, ANEF

CHAPTER 5   **Design-Based Educational Research in Nursing   55**
Anne M. Krouse, PhD, MBA, RN-BC

CHAPTER 6   **Ethical Inquiry in Research in Nursing Education   65**
Barbara J. Patterson, PhD, RN, ANEF

CHAPTER 7   **Managing, Analyzing, and Interpreting Data   81**
Karen H. Morin, PhD, RN, FAAN, ANEF

CHAPTER 8   **Evidence-Based Teaching: Moving Evidence
into Practice   99**
Teresa Shellenbarger, PhD, RN, CNE, ANEF

CHAPTER 9   **Generating Simulation Evidence   117**
Bette Mariani, PhD, RN

CHAPTER 10   **Creating Evidence for Distance Education
in Nursing   131**
Barbara Manz Friesth, PhD, RN and
Anne M. Krouse, PhD, MBA, RN-BC

List of Figures and Tables

LIST OF FIGURES

Figure 1.1   Science of Nursing Education Model   2

Figure 5.1   ADDIE Model of Instructional Design   58

Figure 7.1   The Data Life Cycle   87

LIST OF TABLES

Table 2.1   Summary of Theoretical Considerations in the
Research Process   21

Table 3.1   Selected Potential Funding Sources for Nursing
Education Research   32

Table 6.1   Ethical Issues in Research in Nursing Education   74–75

Table 7.1   Best Practices for Individual Investigators   83

Table 7.2   A Typology of Replication   94

Table 8.1   Journals That Publish Nursing Education Research   102

Table 8.2   Evidence-Based Teaching Practice Goals and Strategies   107

Table 8.3   Research Evaluation Reviews in Nursing Education   110

Table 10.1   Summary of Course Level Definitions   133

Table 10.2   Summary of Program Level Definitions   133

1

Researching Nursing Education

Barbara J. Patterson, PhD, RN, ANEF
Anne M. Krouse, PhD, MBA, RN-BC

As the health care environment becomes increasingly complex, and nurses must be prepared to assume greater responsibility and accountability for the health of individuals, families, and communities in the United States and globally, nurse faculty are challenged to prepare nurses who are ready to meet the demands of this environment. In 2011, the Institute of Medicine (IOM, 2011) called for "nurses to achieve higher levels of education and suggests that they be educated in new ways that better prepare them to meet the needs of the population" (p. 2). Furthermore, the committee called for new models and approaches to nursing education to better prepare students for practice. The challenge, therefore, is to build science of nursing education using rigorous inquiry that advances knowledge and provides evidence to support the design and delivery of education.

BUILDING A SCIENCE OF NURSING EDUCATION

There have been many calls to build the science of nursing education (Broome, 2009; Diekelmann, 2005; Ironside & Spurlock, 2014; Valiga & Ironside, 2012), yet development of a rigorous body of knowledge has been slow because of a lack of funding, a lack of institutional support for faculty research in this area, and the challenges of implementing a robust design for scientific inquiry in educational environments (Broome, 2009; Broome, Ironside, & McNelis, 2012; Ironside & Spurlock, 2014; Valiga & Ironside, 2012). To be able to build the science of nursing education, it is imperative that there is a shared understanding of how it is defined. The following definition emanated from the work of the National League for Nursing (NLN) Task Force on Teaching and Learning (2003):

> The science of nursing education refers to an integrated, comprehensive body of knowledge about how individuals learn to be a nurse or specialist in some area of nursing, how teachers best enhance that learning, how curriculum design and implementation affect learning, how learning and outcomes of the educational enterprise are managed and what skills nurse educators need to prepare graduates for the ambiguous, uncertain, unpredictable, constantly changing world in which they will live and practice nursing. (Gresley, 2009, p. 8)

1

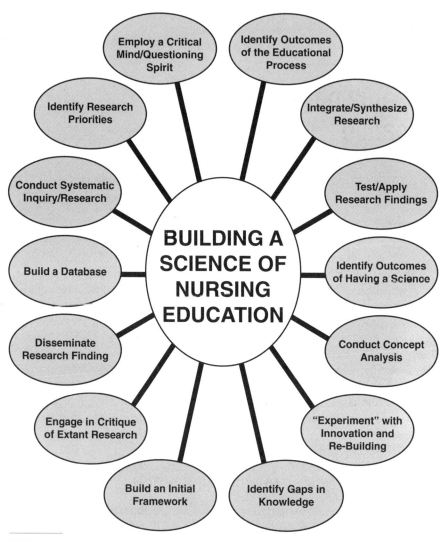

FIGURE 1.1 Science of Nursing Education Model. (Reprinted from *Building a Science of Nursing Education: Foundations for Evidence-Based Teaching and Learning* by C. M. Shultz (2009), New York: NLN. Copyright 2009 by the National League for Nursing. Reprinted with permission.)

The science of nursing education borrows from other bodies of knowledge, such as education, psychology, and the humanities; however, its context, purpose, and relationship to practice make it a unique and discrete body of knowledge. The NLN Building a Science of Nursing Education model (Figure 1.1) depicts the processes involved in building a science. The processes are nonlinear, iterative, and may be simultaneous (Gresley, 2009).

Integral to all of the processes is support for faculty to pursue a program of research focused on nursing education. Administrative commitment to the advancement of the science of nursing education is critical, particularly in the articulation of institutional research priorities, which are reflected in the tenure and promotion process. Additionally, nurse faculty must be committed to improving student learning outcomes through the generation and translation of evidence-based teaching strategies. Investigators must work together to design and implement rigorous multisite studies to move the science forward.

NURSE FACULTY SCHOLARSHIP AS RESEARCH SCIENTISTS

Scholarship involves a deliberative process that includes original research, research that builds on previous work, and a theoretical perspective to frame the research (Kanuka, 2011). A core competency for nurse educators is to engage in scholarship (Halstead, 2007). The scholarship of nurse faculty as clinical practitioners, research scientists, and educators must be focused on advancing the science of nursing and the science of nursing education. To effectively engage in scholarship, faculty must exhibit a spirit of inquiry that embraces and demonstrates the qualities of a scholar: integrity, courage, perseverance, vitality, and creativity (Halstead, 2007). These qualities underpin the work of nurse scientists as they conceptualize, design, and disseminate empirical studies that provide new knowledge to support the teaching and learning of students. Scholarship is essential to nursing education, because "without it our educational practices cannot develop further" (Oermann, 2015, p. 317).

Scholarship and its components have been discussed for many years in the literature, yet the focus of this book is situated in the scholarship of teaching and learning (SoTL), both the process and the product. Nurse faculty want to better understand how students learn and how teaching strategies can maximize student learning. Potter and Kustra (2011) defined the scholarship of teaching and learning as

> the systematic study of teaching and learning, using established or validated criteria of scholarship, to understand how teaching (beliefs, behaviors, attitudes, and values) can maximize learning, and/or develop a more accurate understanding of learning, resulting in products that are publically shared for critique and use by the appropriate community. (p. 2)

This definition encompasses the necessary elements of systematic inquiry, "deliberate, planned, intentional, occurring over time and refined as necessary" (Potter & Kustra, 2011, p. 2) as well as the crucial component of dissemination to the community with public critique. Scholarly peer review by faculty and relevant stakeholders needs to be embraced to advance the science.

The model proposed by Potter and Kustra (2011), the *overlapping magisterial model*, portrays four nested circles with critically reflective teaching at the center, surrounded by evidence-based teaching, theory-guided teaching, and scholarly teaching. Overlapping all four components is the circle of the SoTL. They argue that there are multiple entry points to the SoTL as well as scholarly teaching; it is not hierarchical or linear. The focus of study is teaching and learning phenomena. This model seems to capture all aspects of the SoTL in nursing education, which include critical reflection, evidence-based teaching practice (EBTP), theory, and teaching. It supports multiple research paradigms, sources of evidence, and theoretical perspectives.

An important distinction that Potter and Kustra (2011) put forth in their article is between the SoTL and scholarly teaching. Scholarly teaching is teaching grounded in critical reflection with the goal to improve one's teaching and be an effective teacher. "A scholarly teacher need not be a scholar of teaching and learning . . . for scholarly teaching does not require one to be involved in generating the artifacts used by one-self or any other scholarly teacher" (Potter & Kustra, 2011, p. 5). Excellence in teaching by itself does not constitute scholarship (Oermann, 2015), nor does it make one a credible researcher (Kanuka, 2011).

This distinction is important for the practice of nursing education in that not all nurse faculty will be engaged in research focused on nursing education that empirically con-tributes to a body of knowledge on best practices for teaching and learning. How-ever, being a reflective scholarly teacher with the goal of maximizing student learning is something that all nurse faculty should strive to achieve. Nursing education needs to embrace the development of innovative approaches in learning environments or the use of technology and media to enhance students' learning experiences as a component of scholarly teaching.

In the current higher education climate, research to improve student learning out-comes is a major priority; nevertheless, the value of scholarly teaching cannot be underestimated. The model of the academic researcher/teacher is changing with greater diversity in roles (Kezar & Holcombe, 2015). There remains a critical need in nursing education for both increasing the capacity of the SoTL and scholarly teachers who are intentionally developed, function in a student-centered learning community, and advance the science of nursing education. As noted by Halstead (2007), these activities require a commitment of nurse faculty to lifelong learning and pursuit of career develop-ment opportunities for continued growth as scholars.

KNOWLEDGE DEVELOPMENT FOR THE SCIENCE OF NURSING EDUCATION

It has been argued that educational research is "the hardest science of all" (Berliner, 2002, p. 18). Nurse faculty who have conducted research in nursing education would probably agree with this statement. The challenges that nurse researchers face in examining the problems of teaching and learning are different from those in other sciences, such as chemistry or geology. Likewise, the complexities of education are not analogous to biomedical research and the search for a cure of a specific disease; "there are practi-cal and ethical problems as to whether or how far educational research can replicate controlled methods, even if it wanted to" (Yates, 2004, p. 26). Confounding variables make attempts at replication challenging and may produce inconsistent results. However, it is the power of the teaching-learning environment context and the interactions that provide meaning and understanding for one's teaching practice. For nurse faculty, it is the social interactions among teachers, students, patients, and other involved parties that complicate the science while engaging and stimulating those researchers involved in its advancement.

The complexities of the science of nursing education research and the contribution to knowledge development must be widely acknowledged when the demands to pre-pare competent practitioners is ever-increasing. Rapid technological advancements in both health care and higher education add yet another element to the equation. Provid-ing quality patient care to promote the health of the nation and world requires graduates at all levels to be prepared to lead health care initiatives. Educating future generations of nurse leaders means that educational programs and their faculty need to be at the forefront of learning science. What are the best approaches to teaching, and how does this generation of students learn? Nurse faculty need to question their teaching practice to support a robust science. Flexibility, innovation, and responsiveness to change is crucial for nursing faculty as they teach based on the best available evidence.

Generating the empirical evidence through research is one of the processes needed to build the science of nursing education (Shultz, 2009). The expectation is that the research be conducted in a rigorous, systematic, and ethical manner. Current research doctoral preparation provides faculty with the skills to conduct original research, whereas faculty with the doctor of nursing practice (DNP) degree have the skills to translate the evidence. Both skill sets are necessary to establish best practices in nursing education and contribute to the body of knowledge. Unfortunately, most faculty have limited to no knowledge in the areas of learning sciences and educational theories. Nursing has a professional obligation to strengthen its capacity of nurse faculty with areas of expertise in teaching and learning beyond role preparation as a teacher to achieve the greatest success in obtaining student outcomes.

A Body of Knowledge

A robust substantive knowledge base for nursing education requires nurse faculty to generate the knowledge. Kanuka (2011) advanced the position that those who represent and are experts in a discipline best generate this body of knowledge; she noted, "there are disciplinary differences, with very distinct ways of knowing. These disciplinary differences need to be researched by those whose expertise is in the disciplines" (p. 9). Unfortunately, there exist several barriers to developing and conducting educational research; one significant barrier is the preparation of faculty to engage in educational research (Broome et al., 2012). Given that multiple authors have argued for years that it is time to invest in nursing faculty and nurture those with an educational interest (Benner, Sutphen, Leonard, & Day, 2010; Broome, 2009; Valiga & Ironside, 2012), nurse faculty leaders need to prioritize the reform.

As a professional practice discipline, nurses require a distinctive body of knowledge (Risjord, 2010), and for nurse faculty, educating them requires a body of knowledge about teaching and learning. Nurse leaders need to advocate for the preparation of nurse faculty at the doctoral level so that they may engage in EBTPs and approach inquiry in nursing education from a nursing perspective. Additionally, there need to be plans to develop "high quality, relevant, and cost effective models of nursing education" (Broome, 2009, p. 178). Doctorally prepared individuals focusing on nursing education are in the best position to design, implement, research, and evaluate these models. These steps support the transformation of nursing education and the establishment of a sound knowledge base for best practices in teaching.

Evidence for Nursing Education

Building an evidence base for nursing education cannot occur without rigorous research. Evidence has been conceptualized as "the integration of the best research evidence with theories and concepts about learning, teaching, assessment, and other areas related to nursing education, the teacher's expertise, and the learner's preferences and goals" (Oermann, 2015, p. 304). Multiple studies have examined the evidence that guides faculty teaching practice (Kalb, O'Conner-Von, Brockway, Rierson, & Sendelbach, 2015; Patterson, 2009; Patterson & Klein, 2012). The data from these studies support diversity in evidence and a stronger, more robust empirical basis for teaching practice. Anecdotal experiences and innovative teaching strategies are considered sources of evidence, but they are not the focus of this book.

Although many areas of teaching practice have limited empirical evidence with single-site studies, there are other areas of nursing education where there is a strong foundation of empirical data to guide faculty. Clinical simulation is one area where the body of research evidence is growing strongly and rapidly. Jeffries (2015) highlighted the contributions over the past decade by noting

> there is evidence linking simulation-based curricula to improved patient outcomes, the priority that nurses and other health care professionals strive for when creating and implementing new practices and strategies in education. Overall, simulation pedagogy is growing, maturing, and getting more attention. (p. 359)

These data have provided empirical support for the development of standards by the International Nursing Association for Clinical Simulation and Learning (INACSL) to guide implementation and training for best practices in simulation. Additionally, the NLN Jeffries simulation theory (Jeffries, 2016), a mid-range theory, was developed through theoretical thinking and empirical testing of data collected through multiple simulation studies.

Much of the research in nursing education has focused on how faculty teach and the strategies they use in the classroom and clinical areas. An area of research in nursing education where there are fewer studies and a need for more focused, robust investigations is examining how students learn or the science of learning. By definition, "the science of learning is a systematic and empirical approach to understanding how people learn" (Benassi, Overson, & Hakala, 2014, p. 1). Recognizing this need, one of the 2016–2019 NLN Research Priorities in Nursing Education is to "examine the science of learning in the academic context related to transition mechanisms in health" (National League for Nursing, 2016, p. 3). The intent of these new priorities is to create closer linkages among how faculty teach students, how students learn, and patient care outcomes through robust research designs. Although complex and challenging studies to design, in a practice discipline these connections are critical to advancing the quality of health care.

Theory, Empirical Evidence, and Knowledge

Evidence-based research is necessary in higher education, yet without a theory to help provide an explanation of the complexities of learning, the science will remain at a standstill. Theories are the foundation for knowledge development in a discipline. Broadly defined, theory is "a dynamic system of concepts that provides an organized perspective, explanation, or probabilistic prediction of an aspect of reality or human experience" (Reed & Lawrence, 2011, p. 139). In research, theories provide the perspective and focus for a study from the design and methodology through data interpretation. Likewise, research informs theory. Whether theory generating or theory testing, the relationship between theory and research is a dynamic process, with theories being modified as new evidence is gathered.

Described as the proverbial elephant in the room (Maton, 2006), the extent to which educational theory informs the teaching practice of nursing faculty may be inadequate. Much research in nursing education remains at the descriptive level. In a literature review of the theory base of research in high-fidelity simulation, Rourke, Schmidt, and Garga (2010) determined that only 10 percent of the studies they reviewed made adequate use of theory. Nevertheless, all research has some theoretical underpinning; it just may be implicit. What an investigator selects to study, observe, or measure has a theoretical basis. Theory provides the ontological and epistemological foundations for the evidence (Maton, 2006). Being explicit regarding the theory that an investigator chooses as a framework for a research study is how the science is advanced.

Measurement theory is a good example of the relevance of theory in the decisions that are made in quantitative research studies. As noted by Schmidt (2013), "failure to attend to theory in the selection of measures can limit the utility of findings and call the results of a study into question" (p. 603). The decisions an investigator makes must be grounded in theory; from selecting an instrument, measuring a specific concept, and item generation in instrument development.

Although a detailed discussion of the use of theory in qualitative research is beyond the scope of this chapter, qualitative studies most often start with a school of belief (postpositivist, critical theory, constructivist, participatory) or worldview that informs steps of the research (Creswell, 2016). Creswell suggests that these beliefs shape a study whether introduced at the beginning, emerging in the process, or generated from the data. No matter the research paradigm, without theory, knowledge development and the science of nursing education is hindered with explanation of teaching-learning phenomena limited.

Knowledge Translation and the Translation of Evidence

It is well documented in the evidence-based practice literature that the transfer of research findings into practice is slow and somewhat haphazard (Graham et al., 2006). With the increasing numbers of nurse faculty conducting pedagogical research, the need for translation of empirical findings into one's teaching practice is receiving greater attention. Described as a messy complex social process in the clinical research arena (Bottorff, 2015), knowledge translation of research in nursing education is in its infancy. This process will require collaborative working partnerships among knowledge producers or generators and knowledge implementers or users. A culture of knowing must exist; "communities in which people learn and share knowledge and which are also the sites of knowledge production" (Estabrooks, Thompson, Lovely, & Hofmeyer, 2006, p. 32) are essential to creation of a scientific environment to establish best teaching practices. In the complex higher education setting, this will require recognition of the strengths of the nursing's doctorally prepared faculty and their research skills to achieve optimal student learning outcomes.

Identifying a theory to guide knowledge translation is an important step in the science of nursing education to develop testable interventions. Estabrooks et al. (2006) have argued in clinical practice that "a range of theories is necessary to guide such development and testing [of interventions] at various levels (e.g., individual behavioral, team, and organizational levels)" (p. 29) are necessary to inform the design of implementation research and knowledge translation. With the growth of empirical evidence in the practice of nursing education, investigators are challenged to take the science to the next phase of translation based on theory, but recognizing one theory will probably not fit all contexts. Furthermore, acknowledging the complex nature of the learning environment, Daniel (2012) emphasized that "we need to be open to the potential that recommended pedagogical strategies [based on research findings] may interact with content, other strategies, or competing goals to produce a novel, and potentially undesirable, outcome" (p. 252).

An important element in the knowledge translation process is that the process of translation "occurs in a complex social system of interactions among stakeholders" (Graham et al., 2006, p. 16). Proposed by Graham et al. (2006), the knowledge-to-action (KTA) process is a dynamic model of knowledge translation where stakeholders are incorporated at different points in time. The model includes the full cycle of knowledge translation from knowledge creation to implementation to evaluation to impact. The knowledge producers in nursing education can tailor their research questions to address problems identified by the various stakeholders, whether faculty, clinicians, students, policymakers, or administration, with the goal of making decisions based on empirical evidence. There needs to be an exchange of knowledge among the relevant stakeholders. Additionally, the how and to whom these knowledge producers disseminate the evidence may influence the teaching-learning process and student outcomes.

POSSIBILITIES: CREATING COMMUNITIES FOR LEARNING AND CHANGE

Nurturing and reinforcing a scientific environment within the nursing academic community that emphasizes educational research and best teaching practices in teaching and learning means developing a community based on mutual respect and trust. Progress will be determined through a professional critique of the products of all research endeavors. Individual investigators must be open to dissemination, critique, and revision of their work. Engaging others in discussion of ideas and outcomes of research is how the science advances and the body of knowledge grows. The support from nursing education leadership of investigators whose programs of research are focused on teaching and the science of learning is crucial. It is time to move beyond one type of research being more legitimate than another. It will be through the establishment of a strong sense of community that nursing education will be propelled forward.

Developing a community of scholars to advance the science of nursing education requires the preparation of individuals committed to focusing on the research questions that are of substance and will transform teaching practices (Valiga & Ironside, 2012). These individuals need to be able to think theoretically and design methodologically strong research studies that are more than single site and descriptive. Valiga and Ironside (2012) have argued for a national agenda for research in nursing education that tackles the issues of funding—support for doctoral students and mid-level nursing education researchers who desire or already have a nursing education focus. Another major area of concern as the body of evidence grows will be the translation of research. This is an area of expertise of DNP graduates. Utilizing the strengths of each degree and striving for unity to define a culture of inquiry among all faculty should be the goal.

CONCLUSIONS AND IMPLICATIONS

It is time for nurse scientists to step into the mire of research in nursing education. It is not an easy journey; however, the results of that research have significant implications for student outcomes, nursing practice, and ultimately the health of individuals, families, and communities. The NLN 2016–2019 Research Priorities in Nursing Education (2016) focus on "the generation and translation that builds best teaching and learning practices" (p. 2). Implicit in these priorities is the assumption that nursing education evidence generation and translation is not only important for student learning outcomes but also the health outcomes of patients.

Building and sustaining a culture in which research in nursing education plays a vital role in the profession requires the support of multiple stakeholders. The stakeholders include the nursing faculty, clinicians, administration, students, interprofessional colleagues, and the public. Funding for nursing education is essential. Supporting the faculty whose programs of research are in nursing education is a crucial step in advancing nursing education and the science that underpins it.

Knowledge development requires both knowledge producers and knowledge users. Nurse faculty need to use the evidence to ensure that their students are successful and ready to meet the demands of the complex health care environment. They need to step up to the challenge by reflecting on their teaching practice and the state of the science. These faculty will need the skills to both evaluate and translate the evidence into practice. Educational administrators must support their faculty in this effort by providing education, resources, and mentorship.

The chapters that follow discuss the challenges of conducting rigorous research in nursing education and provide strategies for overcoming those challenges. A well-designed study with attention to rigor throughout the implementation of the study will yield robust results that make significant contributions to the science of nursing education.

References

Benassi, V. A., Overson, C. E., & Hakala, C. M. (2014). *Applying science of learning in education: Infusing psychological science into the curriculum*. Retrieved June 8, 2016, from http://teachpsych.org/ebooks/asle2014/index.php

Benner, P., Sutphen, M., Leonard, V., & Day, L. (2010). *Educating nurses: A call for radical transformation*. San Francisco: Jossey-Bass.

Berliner, D. C. (2002). Educational research: The hardest science of all. *Educational Researcher, 31*, 18–20.

Bottorff, J. (2015). Knowledge translation: Where are the qualitative health researchers. *Qualitative Health Research, 25*, 1461–1462. doi:10.1177/1049732315611266

Broome, M. E., Ironside, P. M., & McNelis, A. M. (2012). Research in nursing education: State of the science. *Journal of Nursing Education, 51*, 521–524. doi:10.3928/01484834-20120820-10

Broome, M. R. (2009). Building the science of nursing education: Vision or improbable dream? *Nursing Outlook, 57*, 177–179. doi:10.1016/j.outlook.2009.05.005

Creswell, J. (2016). *30 essential skills for the qualitative researcher.* Thousand Oaks, CA: Sage.

Daniel, D. B. (2012). Promising principles: Translating the science of learning to educational practice. *Journal of Applied Research in Memory and Cognition, 1,* 251–253. doi: 10.1016/j.jarmac.2012.10.004

Diekelmann, N. (2005) Creating an inclusive science for nursing education. *Nursing Education Perspectives, 26,* 64–65.

Estabrooks, C. A., Thompson, D. S., Lovely, J. E., & Hofmeyer, A. (2006). A guide to knowledge translation theory. *Journal of Continuing Education in the Health Professions, 26,* 25–36. doi:10.1002/chp.48

Graham, I., Logan, J., Harrison, M., Straus, S., Tetroe, J., Caswell, W., et al. (2006). Lost in knowledge translation: Time for a map? *Journal of Continuing Education in the Health Professions, 26,* 13–24. doi:10.1002/chp.47

Gresley, R. S. (2009). Building a science of nursing education. In C. Shultz (Ed.), *Building a science of nursing education: Foundations for evidence-based teaching and learning* (pp. 1–13). New York: National League for Nursing.

Halstead, J. (Ed.) (2007). *Nurse educator competencies: Creating an evidence-based practice for nurse educators.* New York: National League for Nursing.

Institute of Medicine. (2010). *The future of nursing: Focus on nursing education.* Retrieved June 8, 2016, from http://www.nationalacademies.org/hmd/~/media/Files/Report%20Files/2010/The-Future-of-Nursing/Nursing%20Education%202010%20Brief.pdf

Jeffries, P. R. (2015). Signs of maturity . . . simulations are growing and getting more attention. *Nursing Education Perspectives, 36,* 358–359. doi:10.5480/1536-5026-36.6.358

Jeffries, P. R. (2016). *The NLN Jeffries simulation theory.* Philadelphia: Wolters Kluwer.

Kalb, K. A., O'Conner-Von, S. K., Brockway, C., Rierson, C. L., & Sendelbach, S. (2015). Evidence-based teaching practice in nursing education: Faculty perspectives and practices. *Nursing Education Perspectives, 36,* 212–219. doi:10.5480/14-1472

Kanuka, H. (2011). Keeping the scholarship in the scholarship of teaching and learning. *International Journal for the Scholarship of Teaching and Learning, 5*(1), Article 3. Retrieved June 8, 2016, from http://digitalcommons.georgiasouthern.edu/ij-sotl/vol5/iss1/3

Kezar, A., & Holcombe, E. (2015, November-December). *The professoriate reconsidered: What might the faculty look like in 2050?* Retrieved June 8, 2016, from http://www.aaup.org/article/professoriate-reconsidered#.VssxYClGpn4

Maton, K. (2006). *Why theory?: It's not rocket surgery!* Retrieved June 8, 2016, from http://www.karlmaton.com/pdf/2006AAREtheory.pdf

National League for Nursing. (2016). *Research priorities in nursing education (2016–2019).* Retrieved June 8, 2016, http://www.nln.org/professional-development-programs/research/research-priorities-in-nursing-education

Oermann, M. (Ed.). (2015). *Teaching in nursing and role of the educator.* New York: Springer.

Patterson, B. (2009). The nature of evidence-based teaching practice. *Journal of Nursing Education, 48,* 327–333. doi:10.9999/01484834-20090515-05

Patterson, B., & Klein, J. (2012). Evidence for teaching: What are faculty using? *Nursing Education Perspectives, 33,* 240–245. doi:10.5480/1536-5026-33.4.240

Potter, M., & Kustra, E. (2011). The relationship between scholarly teaching and SoTL: Models, distinctions, and clarifications. *International Journal for the Scholarship of Teaching and Learning, 5*(1), Article 23. Retrieved June 8, 2016, http://digitalcommons.georgiasouthern.edu/ij-sotl/vol5/iss1/23

Reed, P., & Lawrence, L. (2011). A paradigm for the production of practice-based knowledge: Philosophical and practical considerations. In P. Reed & N. Crawford Shearer (Eds.), *Nursing knowledge and* theory innovation: Advancing the science of practice (pp. 133–150). New York: Springer.

Risjord, M. (2010). Nursing knowledge. Science, practice, and philosophy. Oxford, England: Wiley-Blackwell.

Rourke, L., Schmidt, M., & Garga, N. (2010). Theory-based research of high fidelity simulation use in nursing education: A review of the literature. International Journal of Nursing Education Scholarship, 7(1), Article 11. doi:10.2202/1548-923X.1965

Schmidt, L. (2013). Keeping the theory in measurement. Journal of Nursing Education, 52, 603–604. doi:10.3928/01484834-20131022-10

Shultz, C. (2009). Building a science of nursing education: Foundations for evidence-based teaching and learning. New York: National League for Nursing.

Valiga, T. M., & Ironside, P. M. (2012). Crafting a national agenda for nursing education research. Journal of Nursing Education, 51, 3–4. doi:10.3928/01484834-20111213-01

Yates, L. (2004). What does good educational research look like? Situating a field and its practices. Berkshire, England: Open University Press.

2

The Role of Theory in Nursing Education Research

Lisa Day, PhD, RN, CNE

Anyone involved in the scholarship of discovery will acknowledge that there are connections between research and theory. Nursing science and the science of nursing education are not exceptions. However, even experienced scientists sometimes have trouble articulating clearly the ways theory and research interact to generate new knowledge in a discipline. Considering that many calls for proposals in nursing education research require the application of a theoretical framework, would-be investigators recognize that this connection must be important. Nevertheless, it sometimes seems like a stretch to link a research question to theory. Although the investigator may not have been thinking of theory explicitly when he or she developed the research question or selected the intervention, theoretical thinking is the foundation to planning and implementing all meaningful research.

Theory provides the ground on which the structure of empirical data collection and interpretation rests and is the glue that holds any study together. Theory is essential to the fundamental design, choice of method, and choice of outcome measures of the study, and a coherent use of theory ultimately will determine whether the study design and findings make sense. Thus, the first step toward a coherent research design, no matter what the research question, is to think theoretically (Meleis, 2012). This chapter offers a definition of theory and describes how theory generally relates to research and how theory is involved in each of four aspects of research design: developing a research question or generating a hypothesis; choosing study variables; and choosing outcome measures. The chapter concludes with three examples from the nursing education literature of different ways theory is used in research.

WHAT IS THEORY, AND HOW IS IT CONNECTED TO RESEARCH?

For nurses, theory can be a confusing and frustrating subject populated by academics who use unfamiliar language and who are far removed from practice. When nurse educators asked students to use theoretical frameworks of theorists like Rogers, Roy, Peplau, or Neuman to plan nursing care for patients, students and faculty alike found that they had to learn a new language. These grand theorists were attempting to make theoretical connections and constructs that could explain all aspects of nursing practice in all possible contexts. The connections between theory and practice have been difficult to support in the all-encompassing way of the grand theorists, and academic nurses have moved to situational and middle-range theories to support their work. Regardless of the type, theory as understood in philosophy and science is an important part of practice and is essential to research.

In the *Encyclopedia of Philosophy,* Hesse (1972) defined theory by contrasting it with law. From the perspective of natural science, laws are observable and operationally definable; theories describe the connections among concepts and ideas that have not yet been observed or cannot be observed. In a textbook on nursing theory, Johnson and Webber (2013) describe theory as "explanation based on speculation" that theorists and investigators expand over time by gathering facts and formulating principles that eventually are accepted as laws (established theory) (p. 11). Thus, the purposes of theory are to take the first step toward understanding the unobserved, to spur us to confirm this understanding using empirical methods, and to create a structure within which one can make sense of empirical (observed) data.

Some of the most abstract theories come from philosophy, where the discussion often involves concepts and phenomena that may never be observed in an empirical sense. In philosophy of the mind, for example, philosophers generate theories about how humans formulate ideas and how the mind interacts with external reality. Taylor (1985) provided an example of this in a paper where he discussed different theories of meaning that draw on connections among language, intentionality, and human expression. Human intentionality and the nature of the mind—how humans move from the physical, objective reality of the external world to understandings and meanings within their minds and vice versa—remain theoretical. Although certain brain functions like metabolism and oxygen uptake with PET scans and functional MRIs can be empirically demonstrated, these laws of human brain function cannot take us all the way to an understanding of human meaning. This leads to competing theories that may seem equally plausible (Dreyfus, 2014; Heidegger, 2008; Husserl, 1999; Searle, 2010; Taylor, 1985).

Like all unobservable or unobserved phenomena, questions of how experiences, perceptions, memory, and language are connected to human meaning start as theoretical discussions. The theorists and philosophers then turn to investigators, who will generate observations through empirical study. Theory is an attempt to explain the unobserved, and research is the attempt to make theoretical connections and constructs observable. As such, research always starts with speculation about unobserved connections or what might be called *theoretical thinking* (Meleis, 2012). Once the theoretical connections are established, the investigator systematically gathers observations that are likely to demonstrate these connections—that is, she or he builds empirical evidence to support the theory; if the observations contradict the connections, the theory is refuted. The investigator then connects each observation or piece of evidence back to the theoretical model. In the next sections, there is a more detailed discussion of how theoretical thinking forms the foundation for generating research questions or hypotheses, selecting meaningful variables and outcome measures, and interpreting research findings.

GENERATING RESEARCH QUESTIONS WITH THEORY

Investigators in nursing education and other fields approach theoretical models in one of two ways: by studying one or more theories and letting the theoretical model generate the research questions, or by generating research questions from practice and searching for an existing theoretical model in which they fit. Either of these approaches requires the investigator to become immersed in theory and theoretical thinking. In the first approach, this is obvious and a natural part of the research. In the second approach, the theory connection can seem arduous and strained unless the investigator has a clear understanding and appreciation of the role of theory in research.

In the example from the philosophical work of Taylor (1985), the theories of meaning come from other philosophers, some of whom he argues against and others with whom he agrees, and he extends these theories with his own thinking. As a philosopher, Taylor is immersed in philosophy of mind and has no shortage of theories to examine, support, extend, or refute through discussion and argument. Similarly, an investigator who is immersed in theories of teaching and learning will be engaged in theoretical thinking and be able to generate new questions from this. But unlike philosophers, an investigator will be motivated to examine these theoretical connections systematically by gathering and interpreting data to construct a model that convincingly demonstrates the connections. In this way, whether the research questions come from theory or from practice, empirical research evolves directly from theory.

Rather than coming from a theoretical perspective, nurses and nurse faculty who are involved in practice often become interested in research when they come upon an interesting question in their practice. For example, a nurse faculty member might notice that students seem anxious when they are in clinical settings and might ask two exploratory questions: what generates anxiety in nursing students, and how does anxiety affect students' learning and performance of clinical work? Or the nurse faculty might notice or hear from students or other faculty that anxiety is causing the students to make mistakes, which might generate a different kind of question: how can students' anxiety be reduced to improve their learning and performance? Having generated a research question from practice, the next step for the beginning investigator is to search the literature. An extensive literature search will include both reports of past research in the area and theoretical discussions broadly related to sources of anxiety, as well as the effect of anxiety on learning and performance. Thus, even the investigator who starts with practice becomes immersed in the world of theory.

The connections between theory and research design most easily are demonstrated in a study that tests an intervention. For example, start with the following question: Does intervention X reduce students' anxiety in a clinical setting and improve their learning and performance? To design a study that gathers meaningful, observable data that might contribute to answering this question, the investigator first has to make explicit the theoretical connections that lead to the original question. For example, what is the source of nursing students' anxiety when they are in clinical settings? How does anxiety impair learning and performance? How does reducing anxiety result in improved learning and performance? And, most importantly, what makes one think that intervention X will reduce nursing students' anxiety? Building a solid research study requires that the investigator answer these questions theoretically before beginning to gather empirical data to support the theory.

MEANINGFUL VARIABLES AND OUTCOME MEASURES

Once the nurse investigator decides on a question to examine and answers the question theoretically, she or he then needs to devise a method for generating data that will contribute to answering the question empirically. This means choosing meaningful dependent variables and deciding on meaningful ways to measure, or in some other way demonstrate, these variables. This also begins with theory. In an intervention study to reduce students' anxiety, X is the independent variable and the dependent variables are anxiety, learning, and performance. Since the purpose of empirical research is to demonstrate the as yet unobserved, there has to be a theoretical connection between the dependent variable and the method of observing, demonstrating, or measuring it.

For example, if one proposed that intervention X will reduce anxiety and then used lower systolic blood pressure post-X as the measure of reduced anxiety, the theoretical connections between anxiety and blood pressure, and between blood pressure and the instrument being used to measure it, for example, a manual sphygmomanometer, will have to be made. Or the investigator can use an established instrument to measure anxiety directly, such as the State-Trait Anxiety Inventory (American Psychological Association, 2016). In this case, the theoretical connections have already been made and there is empirical evidence to support these connections, which are reported as the validity and reliability of the instrument. The only thing left is to make the theoretical connections between the types of anxiety measured by this specific instrument and the types of anxiety likely to be experienced by student nurses in the sample.

The other dependent variables in the example are learning and performance; demonstrating improvements in these areas is more difficult because there are no physiologic markers or established instruments available. This means that the investigator will have to build a theoretical argument for whatever observation or measure she or he chooses to represent improvements in learning and performance. For example, if the investigator uses a teacher's observations and score on a rubric as a measure of a student's performance of a clinical task, she or he will have to make the theoretical links between the rubric criteria and the clinical task, and the theoretical links between teacher observation and quality of student performance. Once these theoretical connections are established, the rubric will need further development, including tests of inter-rater reliability and internal validity, before it will be useful as a measurement tool.

USING RESEARCH TO BUILD AND EXPAND THEORY

When constructing a study to test the effectiveness of an intervention, theory is essential to developing the research question, designing the intervention, and choosing dependent variables and measures. In the example of the study testing an intervention to reduce students' anxiety and improve clinical performance, it is possible to draw on existing, well-established theories that connect anxiety and performance and that suggest possible interventions, dependent variables, and measures. Here are some theoretical connections the investigator makes that are necessary to support the study design: nursing students experience anxiety that negatively affects their clinical performance; the anxiety nursing students experience is typical anxiety that affects their performance in typical ways; and nursing students' anxiety can be reliably and validly measured by established instruments and will be affected by interventions like X that have been shown to reduce anxiety in others. These connections can be made theoretically through argument and can also be supported by empirical evidence that expands existing theory or builds new theory. Exploratory and descriptive studies that provide empirical support for theoretical connections are also ways research and theory are connected.

A study to demonstrate the existence of nursing students' anxiety and to describe it—for example, when does it happen, what precipitates it, what does it feel like, what does it look like, and is it the same in each situation—should precede any intervention study. If there is already an abundance of data that establishes the existence and nature of nursing students' anxiety, the investigator can use these data to support an intervention study. If not, depending on the level of existing data the investigator discovers in the literature review, she or he might start with a qualitative exploration of the phenomenon of nursing student anxiety related to clinical performance or with a quantitative survey to determine the amount and type of anxiety the students experience when they are in clinical settings. Data from these studies will expand the existing theories on anxiety to include specific reference to nursing students' performance in clinical settings.

By integrating theory into their work, investigators are able to design single studies and also develop programs of research over time that will make important contributions to the discipline and science of nursing education. Building the empirical evidence to support theory and deriving theoretical constructs and connections are essential parts of the ongoing development of the knowledge and science unique to nursing and nursing education. Theory sets the boundaries of inquiry by helping the investigator decide what questions to ask, what methods to use, and how to approach data analysis. In turn, the research findings are used to verify, expand, or refute the theoretical constructs and propositions (Meleis, 2012). The more nurse scientists and theoreticians work together to develop strong theoretical bases supported by a variety of evidence for teaching and learning in the unique practice discipline of nursing, the further nursing knowledge and education will be advanced.

ILLUSTRATIVE EXAMPLES

To better understand the role of theory in research, consider the following works published in nursing education journals. Ignacio et al. (2015) noticed that student nurses have a great deal of anxiety and stress related to their clinical performance and asked how an intervention based on mental rehearsal would impact students' experiences. Hamilton, Murray, Hamilton, and Martin (2015) started with the Wellness Recovery Action Plan (WRAP) model for mental health promotion and recovery and built theoretical connections to support this model as a way to reduce stress in nursing students. Levett-Jones, Pitt, Courtney-Pratt, Harbrow, and Rossiter (2015) found that nurse educators know little about the nature and sources of student nurses' anxiety related to clinical placements and asked what the concerns of nursing students are as they prepare for their first clinical experience. Each of these three works—two research reports and one review—highlight different ways research is connected to theory. In this section, these three articles are used as examples of these connections to help nursing education investigators solidify an understanding of the foundational role of theory in science and knowledge development.

Starting With the Question: Finding Theories to Support Research

Like Ignacio et al. (2015), many nursing education investigators start from their practice as teachers by identifying an issue they want to explore, a question they want to answer, or problem they want to solve. The issue may be related to teaching practice or related to the conditions of students' learning. Identifying a problem that might negatively impact learning, such as student anxiety and stress, typically leads the teacher/investigator to search for solutions. Finding a promising solution then leads to an intervention study to measure the effectiveness of the chosen intervention. In the study done by Ignacio et al., the problem the authors identified was students' anxiety that negatively affected their performance in clinical situations; the intervention was a mental imagery exercise; and the outcomes measured were changes postintervention in the students' heart rate (HR), blood pressure (BP), and score on the State-Trait Anxiety Inventory, and in their performance during a deteriorating patient simulation exercise. So how is theory involved in this pre-/posttest intervention study?

In planning a study like this, the investigator should first think theoretically about what makes the question important and what makes the intervention plausible. How are all of the concepts embedded in the research question theoretically connected? For Ignacio et al. (2015), this meant drawing connections between anxiety, stress, performance, and mental imagery. Based on a review of psychological, sociologic, and physiologic theories, these investigators would have found multiple theories proposing connections among stress, anxiety, learning, and performance that travel in multiple directions. For example, anxiety impacts stress, and stress impacts anxiety; stress and anxiety impact learning, and learning can create stress and anxiety; and all of this impacts performance. However, theories such as those of Calvo and Ramos (1989) and Eysenck and Calvo (1992) may seem to disagree with regard to how anxiety influences performance. All of these connections were originally theoretical, and some have since generated empirical evidence to support or refute them. Starting with the theoretical construct that anxiety and stress act as impediments to clinical performance, Ignacio et al. (2015) then further theorized that reducing anxiety would have the opposite effect. Thus, theoretically, an intervention to reduce anxiety and stress should enhance performance. They then chose an intervention likely to reduce anxiety and stress—mental rehearsal. Asking what makes mental rehearsal seem like a good intervention to reduce anxiety and improve performance immerses the investigators in still more theory. What are the theoretical connections between mental imagery and stress/anxiety? The idea that mentally imagining oneself performing tasks will impact a person's actual motor performance was originally a neurophysiologic theory that has since generated empirical evidence to support mental rehearsal as an adjunct to recovery from hemiplegia after stroke and to training surgeons (Nagano & Nagano, 2015; Rao, Tait, & Alijani, 2015). The original theory and subsequent research on the effect of mental imagery on stroke rehabilitation and surgical skills make the intervention plausible in other contexts, but more theoretical connections will have to be made to justify using mental rehearsal as an intervention to reduce anxiety and improve student nurses' performance in complex, anxiety-inducing clinical situations.

Once the theoretical connections between the research question and intervention are established, as well as the desired outcomes, the investigator decides how to measure the outcomes. For the study design to make sense, the measures will have to be theoretically connected to the outcomes, and the outcomes will have to be theoretically connected to the intervention; all of these will have to be theoretically connected to the original research question. Ignacio et al. (2015) chose to measure two physiologic parameters as indicators of anxiety/stress: HR and BP, one survey/inventory of state-trait anxiety, and students' performance scores in a simulation exercise. The theory to support BP and HR as measures of anxiety and stress that are relevant to the proposed effects of the intervention (i.e., reduced student stress and anxiety in clinical situations) draw on physiologic theories of stress that include reference to the hypothalamic-pituitary-medullary axis and the sympathetic nervous system (Hall, 2016). Theoretically, with reduced anxiety and stress, the HR and BP will rise less. The State-Trait Anxiety Inventory is a measure of anxiety that has established validity and reliability, but the relevance of this measure to this study depends on a theoretical connection between anxiety and stress. Measuring students' performance in the simulation exercise completes the theoretical construct of the study by linking reduced anxiety and stress to performance. If the intervention works in the way the investigators hypothesize, students who use the mental rehearsal intervention will have reduced BP and HR, reduced State-Trait Anxiety Inventory scores, and better simulation performance scores than students who do not receive the intervention.

Ignacio et al. (2015) started with a research question—how to improve nursing students' performance in clinical settings—and turned to theory to build a foundation for a particular intervention and set of outcome measures. Drawing from several theories, these authors connected anxiety to stress, and anxiety and stress to performance; they then made a theoretical case for using a mental imagery exercise to reduce anxiety and stress and improve performance. This work of theoretically constructing the research design is the first step toward a coherent research project. The thoroughness with which the investigators approach this step, and the clarity and solidity of the theoretical connections they make, are indications of the rigor and quality of the research design. Had the investigators made the same theoretical connections between anxiety and performance and then chosen an intervention that likely would increase students' anxiety, their design would be incoherent. The theoretical construct would be similarly flawed had they chosen to use a multiple-choice test that measures *knowledge* when the outcome they were interested in was *performance* in clinical situations.

Starting With a Theory: Generating Research Questions From Theory

Many nursing education investigators turn to theory in the way Ignacio et al. (2015) did. After deciding on a question and a method, the investigator seeks out theory to support the research design. This approach works as long as the investigator takes theoretical inquiry seriously and redesigns the study as needed to fit the theoretical constructions as they develop. Another approach to theory and research is represented in the work of Hamilton et al. (2015); however, it is not a research report. Instead, it is a review of the theory behind the WRAP—an intervention to support mental health and well-being described by Copeland (1997). Similar to the mental imagery exercise of Ignacio et al. (2015), the WRAP is embedded in a theory and has generated empirical evidence to support and refute its use in different contexts. By starting with this theory, Hamilton et al. (2015) suggest a structure for their own and others' future research on anxiety, stress, and nursing students' performance.

Starting with a theory before formulating a research question or beginning to design a research project is a good way to keep theory central. Generating research questions from a central theory can also be a path to a coherent program of research that is larger than a single study. Instead of generating one question and then pursuing theories to match, starting with a theory leads the investigator to develop many questions with each successive question building on the last. The discussion by Hamilton et al. (2015) of the theory that underlies the use of the WRAP leads to many research questions related to nursing students' mental well-being that can generate empirical evidence to support or refute the theory. For example, one tenet of the theory that supports the use of the WRAP is that people, external events, or circumstances can trigger negative emotions that lead to increased anxiety and stress. By identifying these triggers and having a self-designed plan to respond to them in a healthy rather than dysfunctional way, students can become more resilient and better able to preserve their mental health. Questions that come to mind related to this construct include the following: What are common triggers for undergraduate nursing students? Do undergraduate nursing students recognize their triggers? What coping strategies do undergraduate nursing students use when confronted with a trigger? Rather than starting with a research project that uses the WRAP as an intervention to support undergraduate nursing students, these preliminary explorations can build support for the use of this intervention with this population.

Building Theory With Research

Rather than starting with a theory, qualitative research methods such as interpretive phenomenology and grounded theory set theory aside and start with an identified phenomenon of interest. This initially atheoretical approach is intentional and purposeful. In describing the phenomenon, the qualitative investigator includes discussions of whatever relevant theories exist, but ultimately the goal is to explore the phenomenon anew and inductively arrive at a new understanding. Unlike a deductive process that starts with a convincing theory, gathers data to support the theory, and then seeks to generalize, an investigator might choose an inductive, qualitative method when the theoretical foundation for explaining a particular phenomenon is inadequate.

The third example is a research work that includes a report of findings of a qualitative study of undergraduate nursing students' concerns as they prepare for their first clinical experiences (Levett-Jones et al., 2015). In a review of nursing education literature, Levett-Jones et al. found a lack of research focused on students' experiences as they anticipate their first clinical experience. Because of this lack, "in-depth understanding of students' specific issues, fears and concerns, strategies designed to support and prepare them may well be inadequate and ill-conceived" (p. 305). These authors sought to add the

TABLE 2.1	
Summary of Theoretical Considerations in the Research Process	
Research Process	**Theoretical Considerations**
Research question/ hypothesis	• What existing theories have addressed this or similar questions? • What parts of a known theory can be investigated empirically or systematically observed?
Method	Choice based on the research question and maturity of the theory: • Exploratory/descriptive (descriptive statistics or qualitative methods) to observe theoretical connections and strengthen the theory • Intervention testing (experimental methods) to build empirical evidence to support interventions that are theoretically plausible • Design of the intervention to advance the theory and refinement of the intervention
Data collection/ measurement	• What are the theoretical connections between the data that the investigator chooses to collect and the research question? • How will this set of data relate to the phenomenon of interest? • What are the theoretical connections between the desired data and the measurement tools chosen by the investigator? • How are the measurements derived by the instruments relevant to the desired data?
Data analysis	• Which parts of the theory do the findings support or refute?

students' voices to the discussion to begin to generate a deeper understanding and theoretical basis for nursing students' clinical performance that is grounded in the students' lived experiences. These authors have moved to an inductive, qualitative method that starts by identifying patterns through observation to draw conclusions that can then contribute to a new theoretical understanding.

Although their findings do contribute to developing new understandings of undergraduate nursing students' anxiety and stress, Levett-Jones et al. (2015) stopped short of a robust qualitative design. As their data collection method, these authors used an open-ended survey question that asked students to write their comments on concerns they have as they prepare for their first clinical experience. They analyzed these data using summative content analysis as part of a larger study that used a mixed methods design. Qualitative methods that use multiple data sources and data collection strategies including interviews, observations, surveys, and document analyses provide a more complete dataset that the research team can then analyze using more rigorous methods. Table 2.1 provides a summary of theoretical considerations that are embedded in the research process.

CONCLUSIONS AND IMPLICATIONS

The title of a poem by Goldsmith (2015) eloquently captures the role of theory in knowledge development: "I Look to Theory Only When I Realize That Somebody Has Dedicated Their Entire Life to a Question I Have Only Fleetingly Considered." Goldsmith's poem reminds us that many of our ideas are not new; we should seriously and deeply look to, and draw from, others' work as we begin our own. Nurse educators immersed in teaching and learning theories such as the experiential learning of Dewey (1966), the social cognitive theory of Bandura (1986), or the social learning theory of Lave and Wenger (1991) can use these theories as starting points in generating research questions. But as is evident in the examples used here to illustrate the connections between theory and research, the work on which investigators draw will not always be teaching and learning theories. When nurse educators generate a research question from their teaching practice, they should turn to a wide variety of theories, including theories of nursing practice and theories developed within nursing education specifically. In this way, investigators in nursing education will be able to design rigorous and coherent studies that will contribute to building the knowledge and science of teaching and learning in the practice of nursing.

References

American Psychological Association. (2016). *The State-Trait Anxiety Inventory (STAI)*. Retrieved May 31, 2016, from http://www.apa.org/pi/about/publications/caregivers/practice-settings/assessment/tools/trait-state.aspx

Bandura, A. (1986). *Social foundations of thought and action: A social cognitive theory*. Englewood Cliffs, NJ: Prentice Hall.

Calvo, M. G., & Ramos, P. M. (1989). Effects of test anxiety on motor learning: The processing efficiency hypothesis. *Anxiety Research, 2*(1), 45–55.

Copeland, M. E. (1997). *Wellness Recovery Action Plan*. Brattleboro, VT: Peach Press.

Dewey, J. (1966). *Democracy and education: An introduction to the philosophy of education*. New York: Free Press.

Dreyfus, H. L. (2014). *Skillful coping: Essays on the phenomenology of everyday perception and action*. Oxford: Oxford University Press.

Eysenck, M. W., & Calvo, M. G. (1992). Anxiety and performance: The processing efficiency theory. *Cognition and Emotion, 6*, 409–434. doi:10.1080/02699939208409696

Goldsmith, K. (2015, April). I look to theory only when I realize that somebody has dedicated their entire life to a question I have only fleetingly considered. *Poetry, CCVI*, 68–82.

Hall, J. E. (2016). *Guyton and Hall textbook of medical physiology*. Philadelphia: Elsevier.

Hamilton, S., Murray, K., Hamilton, S., & Martin, D. (2015). A strategy for maintaining student wellbeing. *Nursing Times, 111*(7), 20–22. PMID: 26477182

Heidegger, M. (2008). *Being and time*. New York: Harper Perennial/Modern Thought.

Hesse, M. (1972). Laws and theories. In: *The Encyclopedia of Philosophy*, volume 4. P. Edwards, ed. London: Collier-McMillan, pp. 404–410.

Husserl, E. (1999). *The essential Husserl: Basic writings in transcendental phenomenology*. Bloomington, IN: Indiana University Press.

Ignacio, J., Dolmans, D., Scherpbier, A., Rethans, J. J., Lopez, V., & Liaw, S. Y. (2015). Development, implementation, and evaluation of a mental rehearsal strategy to improve clinical performance and reduce stress: A mixed methods study. *Nursing Education Today, 37*, 27–32. doi:10.1016/j.nedt.2015.11.002

Johnson, B. M., & Webber, P. B. (2013). *An introduction to theory and reasoning in nursing* (4th ed.). Philadelphia: Lippincott Williams & Wilkins.

Lave, J., & Wenger, E. (1991). *Situated learning: Legitimate peripheral participation*. New York: Cambridge University Press.

Levett-Jones, T., Pitt, V., Courtney-Pratt, H., Harbrow, G., & Rossiter, R. (2015). What are the primary concerns of nursing students as they prepare for and contemplate their first clinical placement experience? *Nursing Education and Practice, 15*, 304–309. doi:10.1016/j.nepr. 2015.03.012

Meleis, A. I. (2012). *Theoretical nursing: Development and progress* (5th ed.). Philadelphia: Wolters Kluwer.

Nagano, K., & Nagano, Y. (2015). The improvement effect of limited mental practice in individuals with poststroke hemiparesis: The influence of mental imagery and mental concentration. *Journal of Physical Therapy Science, 27*, 2641–2644. doi:10.1589/jpts.27.2641

Rao, A., Tait, I., & Alijani, A. (2015). Systematic review and meta-analysis of the role of mental training in the acquisition of technical skills in surgery. *American Journal of Surgery, 210*, 545–553. doi:10.1016/ j.amjsurg.2015.01.028

Searle, J. R. (2010). *Making the social world: The structure of human civilization.* New York: Oxford University Press.

Taylor, C. (1985). *Theories of meaning human agency and language: Philosophical papers 1.* New York: Cambridge University Press.

3

Generating the Research Evidence

Lynne Porter Lewallen, PhD, RN, CNE, ANEF

Sometimes the most difficult part of getting started in nursing education research is just that—getting started. This chapter will offer strategies to begin a nursing education research project, including ideas about finding a focus and turning research interests into a proposal suitable for seeking funding. Examples of nursing education research projects are given for each section.

FINDING A FOCUS

Most investigators in nursing education are faculty members and are involved in many areas of teaching and program administration for which evidence is lacking to support their current practices. One of the issues in research in nursing education is that many of the studies are one-time investigations conducted at a single site. These types of studies often lack the rigor to help advance the science of nursing education. Even small studies are useful in building knowledge, but multiple, sequential studies in the same topical area are more useful in providing evidence for teaching and related areas of nursing education practice, such as program evaluation. Therefore, it is important to spend some time finding a research focus before diving in and starting a project. There are many topics in nursing education that are worthy of investigation. An older inventory of research in nursing education identified 17 domains, including not only academic nursing education topics but also continuing education and patient education topics (Yonge et al., 2005).

As a start, the investigator could consider both personal areas of interest and typical areas of faculty teaching practice. For example, if the faculty member is known for always implementing creative teaching strategies, an appropriate research project might be to study learning outcomes in a group of students using a new teaching strategy compared to students using traditional strategies. Faculty members are often concerned with helping students prepare for the NCLEX®. A research study could focus on exploring the effectiveness of certain strategies in preparing students for success on the NCLEX, investigating variables that are related to success on the NCLEX, or studying strategies of students preparing to sit for the NCLEX after an initial failure. Faculty who teach in the clinical area may want to study student behaviors that lead to clinical success. These are all areas with which most nursing faculty are familiar. Nursing education administrators can also find research ideas in their area of expertise. Examples might be studies related to new faculty retention, the best ways to measure program outcomes, or the best way to schedule clinical courses for student success. Just as clinical nurses are often in the best position to identify important research questions that can have an impact on patient outcomes, nursing faculty are similarly well positioned to identify research questions that will be meaningful in advancing the science of nursing education. Areas of interest and nursing education practice can generate research questions, and this is a logical place to begin.

Another way to find a focus is to go to the literature. It is critical to review the literature on a topic of interest to see what has already been done and where gaps in knowledge exist. This is where to begin to build the science—by extending others' research or replicating studies in different student or faculty populations.

There are literature reviews available on certain nursing education topics, such as simulation, that identify gaps. For example, Cant and Cooper (2010) conducted a systematic review of quantitative literature published between 1999 and 2009 on the topic of human simulation. The studies they reviewed showed evidence that simulation was useful in increasing knowledge and critical thinking; however, samples were small and nonrepresentative, and educational outcomes were assessed in a variety of ways, many of which had limited evidence of reliability and validity. Additionally, many of the variables were measured by self-report rather than a more objective measure. The conclusions from this literature review point to ways the science could be strengthened, and the detail about each study included in review articles such as this is a helpful source of ideas for research questions.

In nearly every research report, there are suggestions for future studies that extend the reported work, which is useful in generating ideas. Replication of well-done studies is important to further the science of nursing education. Since most research in nursing education studies are conducted at a single site, by replicating a study at a different site (or in more than one site), the findings can be extended and the science built. For example, a quasiexperimental study of an interactive strategy to teach undergraduate students about evidence-based practice was conducted in two baccalaureate programs in California. The experimental group showed increased knowledge and ability to use evidence-based practice as compared to the control group, which did not receive the intervention (Kim, Brown, Fields, & Stichler, 2009). This study could be replicated using different levels of students, in schools of different demographic makeup than that of the original study, or in schools in different geographic areas.

Another place to look for research ideas is in agency lists of funding priorities. Later in this chapter, funding sources are discussed in more detail, but most major funding agencies have lists of research areas that they consider a priority for funding. Typically, these areas are broad enough to allow the investigator to take one of several approaches to a research area.

Reading journals that publish articles about nursing education can be a fruitful source for research ideas. As mentioned earlier, research articles in journals typically identify ideas for further research, but non-research articles can also be a source for ideas, as they may describe a teaching strategy or educational issue that lends itself to further study. Most journal articles have contact information for authors, and authors usually enjoy discussing their work with readers. Collaboration can begin through email conversation about an article.

Conference presentations can also be a source of ideas, either from research presentations or those that discuss innovative teaching strategies or other areas appropriate for investigation. Potential collaborators can be identified at conferences. Begin conversations with presenters or with others in the audience about the topic of the presentation. Most nurse faculty are eager to discuss their ideas, and it is easy to network online after the conference is over to plan a joint project. Additionally, using social media such as Facebook™ is an innovative strategy that may be used to solicit research participants or collaborators, or to share ideas (Amerson, 2011). Chapter 9 provides more information on journals and conferences where research in nursing education is published and presented.

Planning the Study/Thinking Innovatively

It is important for investigators in nursing education to design studies that are rigorous. A recent study comparing nursing research focused in the clinical arena to that focused on nursing education found that clinical nursing research was more likely to be externally funded, be multisite, collect objective data, and have a high-level study design such as a randomized controlled trial (Schnieder, Nicholas, & Kurrus, 2013). To improve the quality and fundability of research in nursing education, strategies such as the use of objective measures are recommended, as well as multisite research made possible by collaboration with other nurse faculty within the United States and in other countries as well (Yucha, Schnieder, Smyer, Kowalski, & Stowers, 2011).

Considerations of rigor can vary by study design, but rigor generally refers to designing a research study in such a way that the results can be attributed to the study variables rather than extraneous variables, the sample is representative of the population under study, the variables are being measured in the best available way, and the study procedures are designed to reduce threats to internal and external validity and monitored so that the study is carried out as planned (Polit & Beck, 2016). An example of a study about student preparation for clinical that could advance the science of nursing education, but that is also feasible and could be done with limited funding, will be used to illustrate the concepts discussed in the following section. This proposed study example compares two different methods of student preparation for a day of patient care in the clinical setting. Ways to maintain rigor will be discussed in each section.

Identify the Problem

Clinical nursing education is one example of an area where research is needed. Experts agree that well-designed clinical experiences are critical for effective translation of nursing content into patient care (Benner, Sutphen, Leonard, & Day, 2010). Almost all nursing programs include clinical experiences, so there is no shortage of opportunity for study. The best way for students to prepare for their clinical day is an area in which many faculty struggle. Is it best for the faculty to give students access to all of the information about their prospective patient the day before—should students come into the clinical setting and read the chart, talk to nurses, even interview the patient? Or is it best for students to come to the clinical setting the day of the experience knowing nothing about the assigned patient and first hear about the assignment during report, as an RN would? Or does the best strategy vary depending on the level of the student? These are questions that can make a difference in day-to-day practice for nurse faculty, student learning, and potentially patient outcomes, but often the choice depends on faculty opinion rather than being based on evidence. A study comparing outcomes in two groups of students that prepare for clinical in different ways would provide information on which strategy is best to enhance student learning and performance.

Search the Literature

The first step in designing research about this area would be to search the literature. The purpose of searching the literature is to identify what types of studies have been done in the area and what is known. The studies should be examined first for methodological rigor, considering such factors as the study design, the reliability and validity of the instrument used, and the appropriateness of the analysis. If definitive results were reached, the investigator may be able to use these results as a starting point in planning the next step in the investigation of this area or perhaps replicating the study in a different type of sample. When planning a study, always start with what is known, and build from that. If nothing is known about an area, start from common practice. In the example of methods of clinical preparation, a search of the research in nursing education literature from 2010 to 2016 found only one study related to methods of clinical preparation for undergraduate nursing students (Turner & Keeler, 2015), and this study focused on student perceptions of the preparation method rather than which method resulted in better student preparation to provide nursing care. Given this lack of evidence, it would be appropriate to design a study based on common practice.

Use a Theoretical Framework to Guide the Study

Theoretical frameworks are important to guide nursing education research. Although nursing theories are preferred to guide the generation of nursing knowledge (Smith & Parker, 2015), there are few nursing theories that specifically provide guidance to nursing education practices—theory development and theory testing in nursing education are fertile ground for new research. If no nursing theory can be identified as appropriate for guiding study, theories from other disciplines, such as education, can be useful. Theory can be used in many ways in study development. Theory can be used to guide the entire investigation—the choice of variables, the method of measurement of the variables, how the results are analyzed, and how the results are interpreted in a broader context.

Theory should also be used to design interventions. The sample study used as an example can be guided by the educational theory of constructivism, which posits that students learn best when they are active participants in their learning and can base new learning on previous experiences, and to use new learning in context. Constructivism encourages the use of teaching strategies that engage students actively and help them build on previous knowledge and experience (Utley, 2011). For example, in the case of the study of clinical preparation, constructivism guides the study design with the assumption that that active learning strategies are appropriate to test, and that students should be studied in the real-life context of a clinical nursing unit, and outcomes measured that can be observed in the clinical area. Constructivism can also be used to design the intervention. One of the tenets of constructivism is that learning is enhanced by the use of scaffolding (Melrose, Park, & Perry, 2015), an example of which might be a clinical worksheet to help students identify the important facts to know about a patient prior to caring for that patient. If this theory were guiding the development of the intervention for the study, a clinical preparation tool to help students prepare for the clinical experience, based on their previous learning in related course work, would be used.

Design the Study

When designing a study, there are issues to be considered to ensure rigor. Some of these issues of concern are sampling, measurement, and study procedure. The sample should be selected to ensure representation of the target population. Random sampling is the ideal, but this approach can be a challenge to carry out in nursing education settings. If random sampling is not possible and the study is comparing groups, then random assignment to the groups is best. If this is not possible, then the groups must be chosen to be as similar as possible on variables of interest to the study (Polit & Beck, 2016). This requires the investigator to carefully consider which characteristics of the research participants may have an impact on the variables under consideration.

Another consideration to increase rigor is in the measurement of the variables. If an instrument is used to measure the variables, ideally this instrument has been used before with similar populations and has adequate reliability and validity. Investigator-designed instruments for use in a single study should be avoided. If there is no instrument available for measurement of the study variable, then a pilot study must be done to test the reliability and validity of the investigator-constructed instrument to ensure that the data generated from this instrument will be meaningful to the investigation.

The investigator designs the study procedure to minimize the effects of extraneous variables on the variables of interest for the study. When comparing groups of students, ensure that they have the same level of experience and previous course work. In clinical situations, ensure that the patient populations are similar between the groups so that one patient population would not require significantly more skill to care for than the other. Sometimes differences in groups can be accounted for statistically during the data analysis (Polit & Beck, 2016), but it is best to control for this as much as possible in the study design itself.

Care must be taken in the conduct of the study itself to ensure that the study is actually conducted as planned. This is called *maintaining fidelity* and is a challenge in any study that uses more than one group, especially if the study is also conducted at multiple sites. Some ways fidelity can be maintained are by making sure faculty leading the different groups are aware of the study procedures and are trained to provide the intervention in the same manner, if an intervention is being used. Be sure that data collection is done using the same instruments and at the same time of the clinical day or rotation between the groups.

Using the study example, the investigator acknowledges that usual education practice in clinical preparation is to require students to prepare prior to the clinical day, with some mechanism for them to know details of their patient assignment. A study could be designed to compare this practice to a different approach to clinical preparation, perhaps by having students come to clinical unaware of their particular patient assignment, but providing them with a clinical preparation tool to complete on arrival at the clinical site and giving them a particular amount of time to prepare before beginning care. In a study like this, the investigator would be comparing two approaches to how students prepare for clinical.

For this study, where groups are being compared, the investigator would consider that it is necessary to minimize or account for any differences between the two groups. For example, ensure that the students in each group had the same amount of prior clinical experience so that one group would not do better on the outcome measures simply because that group had more practice preparing for patient care. Ideally, randomly assign students to either the "prepare ahead" group or the "just-in-time" preparation group. Depending on the clinical site or school, this may or may not be possible. To strengthen this study, test this preparation technique in more than one clinical course and in more than one nursing program.

Decide on Outcome Measures

The next step in planning the study would be to decide what outcomes to measure. What is expected to be different in the two groups? How will this difference be measured? It is important to measure outcomes that make a difference in patient care, if possible. Student and/or faculty satisfaction are frequently measured in research in nursing education studies, and although these outcomes might be interesting, they are not as important as outcomes related to actual student performance in the delivery of patient care. Outcomes that might be measured in a study like this are student error rates, student abilities to identify priority nursing interventions using accepted clinical evaluation tools, patient satisfaction with care using standard measures, or quality of the hand-off report at the end of the clinical day using a check-off sheet.

Once the outcome variables have been decided, consider how to measure them. It is best to use reliable and valid measures, if they are available. A literature search may yield measures to use or adapt if they are not exactly right for the study. If a new instrument must be developed, it is best to develop the items using the literature, have the tool reviewed by some experts in the field, and then pilot test the instrument on a group of people similar to those who will be enrolled in the study, prior to using the instrument. This will minimize the risk of not finding differences that are really present because of faulty measurement.

Human Subjects Considerations

Once the study is planned, Institutional Review Board (IRB) approval will be needed if human subjects are involved. Areas to consider when using students as research participants include the following: making sure that participation is voluntary, ensuring that the student's grade is not dependent on participation in the study, making sure that the instructor is not the study investigator, and making sure that incentives are not coercive (Mahon, 2014).

Once the study is approved by the IRB, it is important to plan the steps of the study prior to implementation to ensure the fidelity of the intervention. This is especially important if the study will involve multiple sites or multiple groups in the same site. Fidelity in this context means that the intervention is delivered as intended (Slaughter, Hill, & Snelgrove-Clarke, 2015), and that the study protocol is followed, including the process of collecting outcome measures. If the intervention will run over a long period of time, such as for a whole semester, the nurse investigator should assess the intervention fidelity frequently to identify any issues early and provide answers to any questions about the protocol that might arise. It is not uncommon in multisite research to have different levels of faculty engagement at each of the sites, so the oversight of the principal investigator of the study is crucial (North & Giddens, 2013).

Data Analysis

Once the data are collected, they should be analyzed using appropriate statistical or qualitative analysis procedures. If the investigator is not an expert in either quantitative or qualitative analysis, it is helpful to consult with an expert both when planning the study, to ensure that the procedures and methods are designed to adequately measure the outcomes, and after the data are collected, to help in the analysis and interpretation.

Plan for Dissemination

When the analysis is complete, it is crucial to disseminate the results. The best venue for dissemination is through peer-reviewed publication. Another venue is through national, regional, and local podium or poster presentations. It is wasteful not to disseminate findings if it is possible to do so—it is a waste of the participants' time, the investigator's time, and the funder's money, if funding was secured for the project. Every aspect of the study should be shared to advance the research process and help other investigators learn from experience, whether positive or negative (Resnick, 2014).

SEEKING FUNDING

Many nursing education investigators have ideas for studies that require financial support to conduct, particularly multisite projects. Significant funding for research in nursing education has not been plentiful in the past, but there are more opportunities today for funding. There are a variety of funding sources to investigate for a research in nursing education project.

The National League for Nursing (NLN) has been a leader in funding for research in nursing education and continues to offer both regular research grants and funding specifically for doctoral student dissertations and projects (Duffy, Frenn, & Patterson, 2011). Detailed information about funding can be found at the NLN website (http://www.nln.org/professional-development-programs/grants-and-scholarships), which includes a list of priorities for funding, guidelines and deadlines for submitting applications, and resources to help investigators write successful grant proposals. The NLN has established priorities for funding for research in nursing education, which include discovery and translation of innovative strategies, linking student learning outcomes to sentinel health indicators, and examining patient health transitions from an academic context. Reflecting the core values of the funding agency, all of the priorities contain themes such as leadership, technology,

TABLE 3.1	
Selected Potential Funding Sources for Nursing Education Research	
Organization	**Website**
National League for Nursing (NLN); also has special funding opportunities for doctoral dissertations and projects	http://www.nln.org/professional-development-programs/research/research-priorities-in-nursing-education
Sigma Theta Tau International (STTI)/NLN Grant	http://www.nursingsociety.org/advance-elevate/research/research-grants
STTI/Chamberlain	http://www.nursingsociety.org/advance-elevate/research/research-grants
National Council of State Boards of Nursing (NCSBN)	https://www.ncsbn.org/center-for-regulatory-excellence.htm

ethical codes of conduct, diversity, and partnerships (National League for Nursing [NLN], 2016). NLN funds grants for up to $25,000, as well as smaller grants that are designated specifically for doctoral students. Additionally, NLN partners with other organizations, such as Sigma Theta Tau International (STTI) and Chamberlain College of Nursing, to offer additional funding for research in nursing education.

Another source for funding that offers larger amounts of funding is the National Council of State Boards of Nursing (NCSBN). This organization offers funding through its Center for Regulatory Excellence (CRE), which funds studies that focus on areas of interest to nursing regulators and policymakers. Nursing education is listed as one of the research priorities, and funding is available up to $300,000. Their website provides resources for investigators and answers common questions about writing the proposal. Table 3.1 provides a list of selected organizations that fund research in nursing education.

A variety of other organizations may fund research in nursing education, depending on how the research question is presented. There are several specialty nursing organizations that offer research funding if the study focuses on the target population. A nursing education study might focus on the best ways to educate students to care for that population or the best ways to educate patients in that population. Some nursing programs have access to intramural grants that are designed for faculty teaching in that institution. These grants are often small but can provide funding for small projects or pilot projects.

Conducting a Study With No Funding

Research in nursing education studies, especially small studies, can be conducted without funding, if necessary. Faculty working together can plan and conduct studies in their own nursing program. Collaboration among faculty from different programs can allow larger-scale studies to take place. Some nursing programs may give course release time to allow faculty to engage in the work of conducting a study. By involving undergraduate or graduate students in the study process, some of the work can get done at no cost while the student gains valuable hands-on research experience.

WRITING A RESEARCH GRANT PROPOSAL

Although the idea of writing a research grant proposal can be intimidating, funding can allow the investigator to conduct a sophisticated study that can advance the science of nursing education. The act of writing a proposal can help the investigator to plan every aspect of the study, which can result in a stronger study plan even if the proposal is not funded. It is helpful to ask colleagues to read the proposal before submission. A reader who has not been involved in the writing can often spot missing or unclear areas better than someone who has been involved in the writing from the beginning. Here are some important points to remember as the proposal is written.

Ensure That the Project Aligns With the Funding Agency

There are some important principles to consider when writing a research grant proposal. The first is to assess the organization from which funding is being requested to ensure that it is interested in the research area. Most organizations which fund research will make some sort of statement on their website or provide other materials about the sort of research that is funded. Some organizations have lists of research priorities and previously funded research. If the investigator is not sure if the research idea fits with the priorities or research areas published by the funder, it is worth the time to contact someone from the organization and inquire. Preparing a quality grant proposal is a significant time commitment, so it is critical to ensure that your project fits the priorities of the funding agency so that time is not wasted. When it is clear that the project fits the organization's priority, it is important to make that case in the grant application. Clearly state how the project fits the priority or area of focus for the organization. Grant reviewers respond more favorably to proposals that clearly reflect the priority of the organization.

For example, one of NLN's research priorities for 2016–2019 is the examination and use of technology, simulation, informatics, and virtual experiences on student learning affecting clinical practice (NLN, 2016). A study that would address this priority might examine if students who participated in a simulation experience of a patient developing sepsis would be able to recognize and intervene with such a patient more quickly and accurately than students who learned about sepsis using traditional classroom teaching strategies. In this case, the study examined the use of simulation, which was mentioned in the funding priority, and also linked the simulation learning experience to student learning that could be applied in the clinical practice area. A study that would not completely address this priority might examine student knowledge about sepsis using the two different teaching techniques but not examine how this knowledge affected the care the student delivered in the clinical area.

Read the Directions Carefully

Proposal requirements vary greatly among funders. For many funders, if the directions are not followed, the proposal is not considered, so it is important to read the directions carefully before beginning. Proposal directions highlight areas that the funders will carefully consider, and none of the directions should be ignored. Some areas of variation in proposal directions include the topic headings required; the number of pages allowed; font, spacing, and margin requirements; whether or not appendices are allowed and what they may contain; required elements, such as CV of consultants; submission requirements (electronic or mail); and budget allowances. Some funders require that at least one copy of the submission be de-identified so that reviewers can consider the proposal without knowing the identity of the investigator; for other grants, the identity and qualifications of the investigator is an important element considered in the proposal review.

Ensure That the Proposal Is Methodologically Sound

All of the principles of developing a sound research study discussed earlier in this chapter should be demonstrated in the proposal. The literature review should show evidence of being comprehensive and synthesized, and it should support the need for the study being proposed. It is important to demonstrate how the proposed study fills a gap in the nursing education literature or will extend the science of nursing education (Fitzpatrick, 2012). For example, research in the disciplines of nursing and education has shown that online learning can be as effective as face-to-face learning in knowledge acquisition. If the proposed study examined knowledge acquisition in online education, this literature would be discussed and the case made for why this particular proposed study would extend what is already known.

The theoretical framework should fit the study, and the proposal narrative should clearly demonstrate how the theoretical framework is guiding the research, not just added into the proposal in isolation. The research question must be clear and measurable, and the methods must be appropriate to answer the question. The measurement plans should be appropriate to answer the research question. Valid and reliable measures must be used in quantitative studies. The proposed sample size should be justified, with a power analysis for a quantitative study or a sound rationale for a qualitative study. If possible, the participants should be drawn from more than one site to increase generalizability. When planning an intervention study, a description of the intervention and strategies to maintain the fidelity of the intervention must be discussed in detail so that a study may be replicated. This is especially important if the study will take place at multiple sites or if multiple study personnel are involved in delivering the intervention—this detailed description tells the funder that the investigator has considered all aspects of the study and is likely to conduct it in a way that valid results will be obtained. The data analysis methods should be adequately described and appropriate to the research question and the measures.

Protection of Human Subjects

It is important in any research proposal or any report of completed research to address the protection of human subjects. Plans for IRB consideration of the research are important to document. Some funders require IRB approval (or documentation of exempt status) at the time of submission of the proposal; others require it prior to beginning the study. Much research in nursing education uses students as research participants. Students are typically considered a vulnerable population due to the power differences between students and faculty (Ferguson, Myrick, & Yonge, 2006; Mahon, 2014). Additional IRB safeguards are necessary if any of the research data are to be collected using the Internet (Mahon, 2014). Any conflicts of interest, such as if the investigator has a financial interest in any device being studied, must be disclosed and evaluated by the IRB (U.S. Department of Health and Human Services, 2004).

Budget

Most grant applications have rules about how the funding can be used. Be sure to carefully follow these rules so that the study can be realistically planned. Examples of budget items that are usually allowable would be incentives for participants, fees for electronic survey delivery, and travel costs for data collection. Budget items that are often not allowed are durable goods such as computers or printers that would be used after the study is over or restaurant meals for investigators while collecting data. Some grants will allow part of the investigator's salary to be covered by grant funds; others do not. Grants may allow indirect funds, which are funds that are added to the amount of the grant to support the infrastructure and expenses of the institution in which the investigator is located. Most institutions specify a certain percentage of the total grant requested for indirect funds.

It is also important that the budget include a narrative that justifies the expenses, if required. A detailed justification shows the funding agency that the expenses have been carefully planned and that the requested funding is realistic to accomplish the purposes of the study. An inadequate or missing budget justification shows a lack of attention to detail and may make the grant reviewers question the ability of the nurse investigator to pay attention to the details of the study when funded.

Biosketches and Consultants

Most grant proposals require a biosketch for the nurse investigator. A biosketch differs from a curriculum vitae (CV) in that it includes only information directed toward demonstrating the ability of the nurse investigator to conduct the proposed study. Most funding agencies that require biosketches will specify the desired contents, but typically included are details about the nurse investigator's educational background, a history of research activity (both funded and unfunded), and a list of presentations and publications relevant to the proposed study. Especially important to highlight are presentations and publications resulting from past research, as this demonstrates the ability of the nurse investigator to complete and disseminate research, which is often an important consideration for funders when considering proposals. It is also useful to employ consultants on the project, especially if it can be documented that the consultant brings important expertise to the project that the investigator may be lacking. This indicates that the nurse investigator is clear about his or her own strengths and weaknesses, has thought through the skills needed to complete the proposed research, and has assembled a team that together have the necessary skills.

Grant Reviews

Representatives of the funding agency review the grant proposals. The reviewers may be volunteer peer reviewers, or they may be employees of the funding agency. Some agencies will offer review comments to the nurse investigator, especially if the proposed study is not approved for funding. These comments can be helpful in revising the study plan to submit for future funding. Whether a study is funded or not, strengthening a study design based on feedback prior to conducting the study can contribute to best practices in research in nursing education.

CONCLUSIONS AND IMPLICATIONS

Research in nursing education is needed to advance our science and allow us to educate students from a base of evidence. Methodologically sound studies can provide evidence for teaching and support best practices. Multiple areas in nursing education are ripe for investigation. Small studies can be done without funding, but funding for research in nursing education is becoming more available. Taking the time to design rigorous studies is crucial to advancing the science of nursing and nursing education. Patient care outcomes ultimately depend on best practices in nursing education.

References

Amerson, R. (2011). Facebook: A tool for nursing education research. *Journal of Nursing Education, 50*, 414–416. doi:10.3928/01484834-20110331-01

Benner, P., Sutphen, M., Leonard, V., & Day, L. (2010). *Educating nurses: A call for radical transformation*. San Francisco: Jossey-Bass.

Cant, R. P., & Cooper, S. J. (2010). Simulation-based learning in nurse education: Systematic review. *Journal of Advanced Nursing, 66*, 3–15. doi:10.1111/j.1365-2648.2009.05240.x

Duffy, J. R., Frenn, M., & Patterson, B. (2011). Advancing nursing education science: An analysis of the NLN's grants program 2008–2010. *Nursing Education Perspectives, 32*, 10–13.

Ferguson, L. M., Myrick, F., & Yonge, O. (2006). Ethically involving students in faculty research. *Nurse Education Today, 26*, 705–711.

Fitzpatrick, J. J. (2012). Building the science of nursing education research. *Nursing Education Perspectives, 33*, 291.

Kim, S. C., Brown, C. E., Fields, W., & Stichler, J. F. (2009). Evidence-based practice-focused interactive teaching strategy: A controlled study. *Journal of Advanced Nursing, 65*, 1218–1227. doi:10.1111/j.1365-2648.2009.04975.x

Mahon, P. Y. (2014). Internet research and ethics: Transformative issues in nursing education research. *Journal of Professional Nursing, 30*, 124–129. doi:10.1016/j.profnurs.2013.06.007

Melrose, S., Park, C., & Perry, B. (2015). *Creative clinical teaching in the health professions*. Retrieved June 9, 2016, from http://epub-fhd.athabascau.ca/clinical-teaching/

National League for Nursing. (2016). NLN research priorities in nursing education 2016-2019. *NLN Professional Development Programs*. Retrieved June 9, 2016, from http://www.nln.org/professional-development-programs/research/research-priorities-in-nursing-education

North, S., & Giddens, J. (2013). Lessons learned in multisite, nursing education research while studying a technology learning innovation. *Journal of Nursing Education, 52*, 567–573. doi:10.3928/01484834-20130313-02

Polit, D. F., & Beck, C. T. (2016). *Nursing research: Generating and assessing evidence for nursing practice* (10th ed.). Philadelphia: Wolters Kluwer/Lippincott Williams & Wilkins.

Resnick, B. (2014). Dissemination of research findings: There are NO bad studies and NO negative findings. *Geriatric Nursing, 35*, S1–S2. doi:10.1016/j.gerinurse.2014.02.012

Schnieder, B. S., Nicholas, S., & Kurrus, J. E. (2013). Comparison of methodologic quality and study/report characteristics between quantitative clinical nursing and nursing education research articles. *Nursing Education Perspectives, 34*, 292–297.

Slaughter, S. E., Hill, J. N., & Snelgrove-Clarke, E. (2015). What is the extent and quality of documentation and reporting of fidelity to implementation strategies: A scoping review. *Implementation Science, 10*, 129. doi:10.1186/s13012-015-0320-3.

Smith, M. C., & Parker, M. E. (2015). *Nursing theories and nursing practice* (4th ed.). Philadelphia: F. A. Davis.

Turner, L., & Keeler, K. (2015). Should we prelab? A student-centered look at the time-honored tradition of pre-lab in clinical nursing education. *Nurse Educator, 40*, 91–95. doi:10.1097/NNE.0000000000000095

U.S. Department of Health and Human Services. (2004). *Financial relationships and interests in research involving human subjects: Guidance for human subject protection*. Retrieved June 9, 2016, from https://www.abramsoncenter.org/media/1181/dhhs-final-guidance-document-on-financial-relationships-in-research-involving-human-subjects.pdf

Utley, R. (2011). *Theory and research for academic nurse educators: Application to practice.* Sudbury, MA: Jones & Bartlett.

Yonge, O. J., Anderson, M., Profetto-McGrath, J., Olson, J. K., Skillen, D. L., Boman, J., et al. (2005). An inventory of nursing education research. *International Journal of Nursing Education Scholarship, 2*(1), Article 11. Available at http://www.bepress.com/ijnes/vol2/iss1/art11

Yucha, C. B., Schnieder, B. S., Smyer, T., Kowalski, S., & Stowers, E. (2011). Methodological quality and scientific impact of quantitative nursing education research over 18 months. *Nursing Education Perspectives, 32*, 362–368.

4

Measuring Educational Concepts

Darrell Spurlock, Jr., PhD, RN, NEA-BC, ANEF

Building a robust science of nursing education requires that researchers be able to study phenomenon of interest to the discipline in increasingly complex ways over time. Systematic inquiry into a phenomenon (or *construct*) of interest to nursing education can take many forms. In some cases, early exploration of constructs occurs through qualitative investigations that seek to identify, define, or clarify the parameters or characteristics of a construct. In other cases, a phenomenon may have been defined already, but new theories or questions have emerged, necessitating further inquiry. In any case, a fundamental requirement for continuing knowledge development is the ability to *measure* the construct of interest. In social science research traditions, measurement can be defined as the act of determining the characteristics, dimensions, or amount of a construct (Thorndike & Thorndike-Christ, 2011). Educational measurement often refers to the process of measuring knowledge, attitudes, values, beliefs, and abilities relevant to the educational process.

The purpose of this chapter is to provide practical guidance in support of rigorously measuring educational concepts in nursing education research. Given the broad scope of the topic of educational measurement (there are entire doctoral degree programs focused on educational measurement!), this chapter will focus on providing an overview of measurement approaches and measurement theory, principles of evaluating and selecting measures for nursing education research, the process of instrument/measure development, and some key measurement-related considerations that support development of a robust science of nursing education. Although a wide range of disciplinary perspectives have influenced measurement practices in nursing education research, this chapter gives strong preference to the approaches from psychology and education that have had the strongest influence—and with which nursing education researchers are likely to be most familiar. Other perspectives, especially those increasing in popularity and acceptance, are discussed when appropriate.

MEASUREMENT AND MEASUREMENT THEORY

Several definitions are in order to provide coherence throughout the rest of this chapter. It should be noted that most of the following terms have no universally agreed-upon definition, and as such, readers may encounter slightly different definitions when referencing a variety of sources within and outside the nursing literature. Nursing educators and researchers are typically well acquainted with *nursing theory,* having studied such theorists as Florence Nightingale, Hildegard Peplau, and Virginia Henderson in undergraduate through doctoral programs. Many of the terms noted are commonly used in nursing theory, but the conventions of their use in educational and psychological research can vary slightly. Readers are encouraged to explore more detailed resources on the theoretical basis of nursing, such as McEwen and Wills (2014) or Chinn and Kramer (2014). Those interested in exploring perspectives from the philosophy of science may like the comprehensive review provided by Martin, Sugarman, and Slaney (2015).

Measurement Definitions

Mentioned in the introductory section, a construct is an abstract mental representation that is often inferred from observable events or behaviors (DeVellis, 2012). Although many would disagree about the appropriateness of doing so, the term *construct* is often used interchangeably with terms such as *phenomenon, concept,* or *variable.* Constructs vary in their level of abstraction. For example, *speed* or *length* is less abstract than *knowledge* or *understanding.* By extension, constructs can be measured more or less directly, depending on the level of abstraction. Whereas the speed of completing a given task is directly measurable using a variety of methods, the *accuracy* or *completeness* — or to use an example from nursing, completing the task *safely* — is less directly measured and is therefore inferred, based on rules and principles set out by the researcher.

Educational and psychological researchers often use the term *latent trait* to describe a human characteristic or trait that is unobservable using existing methods and thus requires measurement-based inferences. Examples of latent constructs include knowledge, ability, personality, and critical thinking, among others. These constructs cannot be directly observed, but their existence is inferred through the administration of tests, assessments, and other measures. Performance on the measure indicated by a score or ranking is theorized to be causally related to the amount of the underlying latent constructs an individual possesses. In a general example, a higher score on a measure of confidence indicates higher levels of confidence, and so on.

The act of *measurement* is an attempt to represent the construct of interest using *indicators* of the construct (Thorndike & Thorndike-Christ, 2011). Indicators are formalized into *measures* and *scales* and *instruments,* terms often used interchangeably, including in this chapter. Measures or instruments are comprised of *items* that, when combined with the numerical values contributed from other items, produce *scores* that quantitatively represent the amount or some other characteristic of the underlying construct. These terms are used with instruments as diverse as attitude scales, multiple-choice exams, and behavioral observation tools. One important note to make here is in the use of the term *scale.* Educators and researchers often use this term to refer to the entire measurement tool or instrument (e.g., *anxiety scale*), but the term also has meaning in describing the units of measurement used at the individual item level. For example, when asking respondents to a questionnaire item to rate the extent to which they agree with the statement made in the item, they can often provide this rating on a 5-point or 7-point scale. Thus, *scale* can refer to an entire measurement instrument comprised of many items, or it can refer to the units of measure used for an individual item. Last, as described earlier, *educational measurement* refers to the process of measuring knowledge, attitudes, values, beliefs, abilities, and other constructs relevant to the educational process.

Purposes of Measurement

Thorndike and Thorndike-Christ (2011) note that the practice of educational and psychological measurement has developed to support decision making by educators, researchers, leaders, and others about the people being measured. The first consideration when approaching educational measurement is to evaluate the purpose of measurement, and more specifically, the purpose or intended use of an individual measure or instrument. An individual measure can have several purposes or only one. Typically, the creators of a measure will clearly define the purpose of the measure. This can sometimes be quite theoretical in nature or could be much more practical. For example, Spurlock and Wonder (2015) created a measure of evidence-based practice (EBP) knowledge for nurses in the form of a multiple-choice test. Although multiple-choice tests can be used in several ways, the authors clearly stated that the measure was not designed for decision making about individuals but rather was designed for use in research and educational program evaluation contexts.

Polit and Yang (2016), although focused on measurement in health research, describe three main purposes of measurement, which are wholly relevant to educational measurement: discriminative, predictive, and evaluative. *Discriminative* measures are used to assess differences between groups or individuals. An example of a discriminative educational measure is a norm-referenced achievement test. These tests, often supplied by test vendors, aim to measure individual mastery of a specified knowledge content area and provide normative comparisons of the individual to a large sample of examinees (usually called the *norming sample*). Such tests provide at least an individual score and a percentile score, reflecting where the individual score falls on the continuum of scores from the larger norming sample.

Predictive measures are also quite common in education, specifically in nursing education. To continue with the previous example, an achievement test can also function as a predictive measure if scores from the test, through extensive research, have been correlated with an outcome such as success in college, success on a licensing examination, or success in employment roles. Nurse educators and nursing education researchers are generally quite familiar with the wide range of tests, which claim to predict a student's success on the National Council Licensure Examination—Registered Nurses (NCLEX-RN®).

Last, *evaluative* measures are used to evaluate the effectiveness of an intervention or treatment. An educational example familiar to many nurse educators is measures of critical thinking. Critical thinking is often an important outcome of higher education degree programs, including those in nursing. Measures of critical thinking such as the California Critical Thinking Skills Test (CCTST; Insight Assessment Inc., 2015) are often used to measure critical thinking skills before, during, and after a degree program designed to facilitate development of those skills. In this way, the purpose of the assessment is to evaluate the causal relationship between the educational program and the development of desirable higher-order, critical thinking skills.

Thorndike and Thorndike-Christ (2011) describe several common purposes of measurement in terms of the kinds of practical, applied decisions made in response to measurement. *Instructional* or *curricular* decisions involve making inferences about the effectiveness of instructional methods and the curriculum within which the instruction is a component. These decisions can be at level of the individual, the class, the school, or even across programs and sites. *Selection* decisions, such as when selecting a new employee or admitting a student to an educational program, are often heavily based on information derived from measures. Similarly, *placement* and *classification* decisions involve using measurement data to stratify candidates based on ability, aptitude, or appropriateness to a role or type of work. The last type of decisions are *personal* decisions. These decisions help individuals understand their own strengths, opportunities for growth, and other characteristics in support of personal choices in career, college, or relationships. In practical applications, measures can be designed to serve several purposes, as the preceding examples illustrate.

Types of Measures

There are many ways to classify measures. In the previous section, measures were classified based on their intended purposes or functions. Another way to classify measures is based more on the technical form of the measure than its intended purpose. Educational measures can be divided into four main types based on how information for the measure is elicited: self-report, observation, psychometric, and tests (examinations). *Self-reports* encompass a wide range of measures that rely on individuals providing responses directly to the items on a scale. Examples of self-reports can include measures and scales addressing feelings and moods, career interests, values, beliefs, and attitudes. Self-report measures are often the easiest to locate and administer but also have several well-documented limitations, mainly centered on cognitive bias and its effect on the accuracy of self-reports. A complete discussion of these limitations is beyond the scope of this chapter, but to provide one example, nurse educators often rely on student self-reports of competence in the clinical setting, perhaps as part of a dyadic evaluation (of which the faculty member is the other half). Bowman (2010) examined the correlations between self-reports and objective measures of learning and development in areas such as critical thinking, personal ethical development, and academic achievement among 3,072 college students. He found correlations of between 0 and .2 between self-reported and objective measures of learning and development, calling into serious question the validity of students' self-reports of learning or achievement. Further, a recent metasynthesis of 22 meta-analyses (Zell & Krizan, 2014) found a mean correlation of only .29 between self-reports and objective measures of ability across a wide range of performance domains, including athletic ability, medical/clinical skills, and academic achievement. Dunning and Helzer (2014) extend this by examining correlation coefficients to include measures of bias, which when considered further diminish the extent to which educators and researchers should rely on self-assessments when more direct measures are available.

Observational measures come in many forms but generally involve direct observation by another person with recording of information according to the design of the observational measure. Examples of observational measures include performance rubrics, functional evaluation of physical capacity measures, checklists, and behavior rating scales. To be most useful in research contexts, well-designed observational measures generally must demonstrate high *inter-rater reliability,* which is the ability to produce consistent measurements even when the measures were taken by different raters.

The next type of measure, the *psychometric* measure, is a broad class of measures that are designed to measure a psychological construct using strategies and techniques not obvious to the subject completing the measure, compared to self-reports where the purpose of the instrument or scale is more readily discernible. Some would argue that the distinction between a self-report measure and a psychometric measure is artificial, as many psychometric measures involve self-report. This critique is not without merit, but the distinction is worth making for the sake of understanding the very different theoretical basis underlying each type of measure. Two classic types of psychometric measures, both of which gave rise to the term *psychometric,* include personality assessments and intelligence assessments. These types of measures usually involved completing a large number of theoretically derived items that then form a composite or index score on one or more traits. An example psychometric instrument with which readers may be familiar is the Myers-Briggs Type Indicator (MBTI) inventory, used to identify one's preferences along several dimensions of personality. Although popular, the validity and reliability of the MBTI has been questioned (Pittenger, 2005).

The last major type of education measure is the *test,* also known as an *examination* in classroom settings. Indeed, like many other topics in this chapter, even textbooks devoted to the subject of testing and test development are quick to note the limitations of what can be covered in a single volume. Several excellent resources for nurse educators include the psychology and education-oriented text by Thorndike and Thorndike-Christ (2011) and the nursing education-oriented text by McDonald (2014). There are several main types of tests, including aptitude, achievement, and performance tests. Thorndike and Thorndike-Christ (2011) note that aptitude tests are designed to measure a person's cognitive ability, with the intention of being able to predict future performance. There are a multitude of these types of measures, with as many different theories of intelligence and cognitive ability serving as the basis for the measures. In some ways, an aptitude measure could be more accurately thought of as a psychometric measure than a test, but this typology is mainly a matter of personal preference. Achievement tests, discussed earlier in the chapter, are designed to measure existing knowledge and understanding—what a person has already learned and, in some cases, how well he or she can apply that information in novel situations. In this way, most classroom exams are achievement tests. The NCLEX-RN is a type of achievement test in that it measures the knowledge necessary to provide safe nursing care at the entry level of professional nursing practice. Commercial test vendors provide a range of standardized achievement testing products to nursing education programs, usually in alignment with national curriculum and NCLEX-RN content standards. The term *standardized* implies that the test has established (and published) normative data so that comparisons can be made across individuals, groups, and time.

Measurement Theories

There are two main theories of measurement with which nursing education researchers should familiarize themselves. The first, *classical test theory* (CTT; also sometimes called *classical measurement theory* [CMT]), has a long history and is well understood and accepted across multiple disciplines, including nursing. Downing (2003) suggests that CTT can be summarized in one statement: "Every test score is composed of two components: true score and error" (p. 740). The equation used to represent this statement is depicted as $X = T + e$, where X is the true score, T is the observed score, and e represents measurement error. Essentially, CTT suggests that there exists a true score that is composed of the score observed or obtained during testing and some amount of measurement error. Although the observed score is easily understandable, one challenge with CTT is that the error term is a composite, undifferentiated term where all sources of error, including poor test construction, differences in scores across groups and across time, and any other sources of error, are all combined into a single error term (DeVellis, 2012). Original conceptions of CTT suggested that error be examined through the lens of reliability, defined by DeVellis as "the proportion of variance attributable to the true score of the latent variable" (p. 31). DeVellis depicts this as *reliability = true score/observed score*. Given this model, measures that are highly reliable are thought to have a low proportion of error, reflecting scores that are closer to the actual true score.

Reliability can be assessed in a variety of ways, but most commonly, Cronbach's alpha is the metric of choice in educational research. Other methods for evaluating the reliability of a measure include test-retest, parallel forms, and split-half techniques. Cronbach's alpha is a measure of the internal consistency of responses to scale or measure and is depicted as a value between 0 and 1.0, where 0 indicates no consistency or pattern to responses and 1.0 indicates no variation in the response data. In most cases, when there is just one underlying construct being measured by a scale, strong internal consistency in responses is desired. A generally held view is that alpha values of .70 to .90 are desirable, with lower values representing lower levels of internal consistency and values greater than .90 likely indicating redundancy of items on the scale.

There are many critiques of Cronbach's alpha as a measure of reliability, mainly focusing on (a) how easy it is manipulate, (b) that it is a lower bound (conservative) estimate of reliability, and (c) that it is highly tied to the specific sample of subjects to whom the measure was administered. On the first account, because Cronbach's alpha is sensitive to both the number of items on the scale and the number of responses to those items (provided by subjects), to increase alpha, one generally need only to increase one or the other of those factors. Thus, if pilot testing of a 10-item scale among a sample of $N = 60$ subjects produces an alpha of .62, by either adding additional items to the scale or increasing the number of subjects providing responses, it may be possible to achieve alpha levels higher than the desired level of .70. In this scenario, poorly performing items could remain on a scale when the better choice would have been to revise or improve the items based on a more extensive item analysis. The second criticism is highly technical in nature, but in sum, the underlying mathematics of Cronbach's alpha tends to underestimate reliability in certain situations. Over the years, several adjusted methods of calculating alpha have been proposed and can be explored further in Sijtsma (2009), for those interested in this topic. The last criticism of Cronbach's alpha, dealing with the sample-dependent nature of the metric, is actually a critique of CTT more generally. Under CTT, reliability estimates are highly bound to the particular subjects providing responses to the scale. Because in CTT there is no distinction made between sources of error attributable to the subjects versus to the items themselves, as Downing (2003) notes, the two sources of error are hopelessly confounded. Being unable to easily disentangle how an item performs across time and among different subjects from how a particular group of subjects performs at a given time is the source of the confounding described by Downing.

The other major measurement model of interest to nursing education researchers, *item response theory* (IRT), seeks to address the limitations of CTT. IRT is an organizing framework for a family of techniques whose main advantage over CTT is that both the trait being measured and the characteristics of the respondents are considered simultaneously on a logarithmic scale where the latent trait is depicted along the x-axis and the probability of a given response is depicted along the y-axis. (*Note:* Explanations of IRT vary across reference sources, with a tendency to use language consistent with the particular use of IRT in question. For example, if IRT is being used to develop an examination, the term *ability* may be substituted for *latent trait.*) DeVellis (2012) describes the main goal of IRT as to establish information about scale items that is independent of the subjects completing them, using a physical measurement analogy to illustrate the IRT approach. Like a physical measure such as weight, where 15 pounds means the same thing no matter the characteristics of the object being weighed, IRT seeks to measure the amount of the latent trait no matter the characteristics of the subject being measured. Because IRT focuses more strongly on individual item characteristics rather than the whole scale, such as is the case in CTT, with a sufficiently heterogeneous sample of subjects representing a wide continuum or range of the underlying latent trait, it becomes possible to overcome the problem of sample dependency present in CTT. Although there are similarities between CTT and IRT, researchers unfamiliar with IRT may find the terms and technical requirements of IRT to be more complex than CTT. Readers seeking a more complete explanation and comparison between CTT and IRT/Rasch are encouraged to review either De Champlain (2010) or DeVellis (2012).

EVALUATING AND SELECTING MEASURES

Often, one of the earliest steps in the research process is to locate, evaluate, and select instruments or scales that will enable the researcher to answer the research questions. Although this may seem like a straightforward task, there are a variety of factors to consider. A preliminary step in this process is to locate available and appropriate measures. There are four main sources that nursing education researchers may want to consider, presented here in the order in which the source should be consulted. The first are electronic databases, some of which specialize in collating information on measures, instruments, and scales, such as the Health and Psychosocial Instruments (HAPI) and PsychTESTS databases. These proprietary databases (and others like them) are generally available through university libraries and are searched much like regular scholarly databases or indices. The results are generally in the form of abstracts for original instrument development papers with full-text access to the paper depending on the individual university's access to the journal or source in which the paper appeared. Some of these specialized databases may be just subsets of larger scholarly databases, and therefore the information will be similar or identical between the specialized database and the more general one.

The usefulness of such specialized databases has become more limited due to the development of more robust searching functionality within general scholarly databases. For example, the Education Resource Information Center (ERIC) is a specialized education-focused index managed by the U.S. Department of Education. It can be searched using limiters so that only instrument or measurement papers are returned in the search results. The same techniques can be applied to other scholarly databases/indexes such as PubMed and the Cumulative Index of Nursing and Allied Health Literature (CINAHL), databases with which nursing education researchers are familiar. Because access to these databases is available through several commercial vendors, the options for searching and retrieving selected papers varies widely.

The second major source for locating measures is in print-based or electronic compendia of research instruments. There are several varieties of these, including the print-based *Mental Measurements Yearbook* (Carlson, Geisinger, & Johnson, 2014) and the electronic Test Link database provided by the Educational Testing Service (ETS; Educational Testing Service, 2015). The *Mental Measurements Yearbook* focuses heavily on several dozen psychological instruments, whereas the ETS Test Link database provides information on more than 25,000 education-oriented measures applicable to education across the life span. Because the range of topics of interest to nursing education researchers is so broad, instruments may also be found in health-oriented volumes released on an irregular basis.

A third source of instruments is professional and research organizations. Examples include the Medical Outcomes Trust and the RAND Corporation. These nonprofit research organizations have developed or manage rights for a wide range of research and survey instruments, many of which could be of interest to nursing education researchers. Access and searching is available online through pages on the organizations' websites.

The fourth main source for finding and locating instruments useful for nursing education research is the Internet. Many authors of instruments and measures may retain control of the distribution and use of the measure, making the tool available only by request through a dedicated website or the author's professional website. This does not mean that there are no published data to evaluate the usefulness of the instrument in a given study, but to be sure, an increasing number of tools are available only through the instrument authors' websites. Oftentimes, this site will be a university-supplied subdomain for a faculty member who has developed a measure, but just as often it may be a page designed and controlled by the instrument author. As DeVellis (2012) noted, these pages are often fleeting in nature and may not be maintained over the long run, so researchers must consider this when selecting measures.

Once a measure has been located, prior to selecting the measure for use, the researcher must evaluate the instrument along several dimensions for fit, appropriateness, and quality. Although there are no true gold standard requirements or even standardized procedures for instrument development, several guidelines are available to assist nursing education researchers in evaluating the quality and sufficiency of psychometric reporting for commonly used scales and measures. Perhaps the most general, recent, and applicable to nursing education are provided by Streiner and Kottner (2014) and are an extension of the Guidelines for Reporting Reliability and Agreement Studies (Kottner et al., 2011). While providing some guidance on the process of instrument development, the guidelines are most helpful in framing the expectations for reporting in instrument development studies. The authors provide section-by-section guidance on the suggested content of instrument development reports, covering topics such as adequately describing the sample, the item development process, common statistical procedures that provide evidence of reliability, and addressing issues of ethics and funding disclosures. Novice and experienced researchers would do well to develop a checklist based on Streiner and Kottner's work and implement this in evaluating potential instruments for use in a study. Other authors (e.g., see Artino, La Rochelle, Dezee, & Gehlbach, 2014; Barry, Chaney, Piazza-Gardner, & Chavarria, 2014; Barry, Chaney, Stellefson, & Chaney, 2011; Lucas, Macaskill, Irwig, & Bogduk, 2010), in offering practical advice on instrument and scale development, provide similarly valuable information for the instrument evaluation process. Although not directed at educational researchers, the Patient Reported Outcome Measurement Information System (PROMIS®) Instrument Development and Validation Scientific Standards (Patient-Reported Outcome Measurement Information System, 2013) provide extensive guidelines and technical standards for instrument development, much of which is applicable—and perhaps, aspirational—to educational measures and instruments. The PROMIS guidelines address conceptual model development, item generation, testing and instrument formatting, establishing validity and reliability evidence, and interpretation and translation of instruments. All of these topics are important to instrument development, no matter the subject of the measure.

From a universe of possible considerations a researcher must make in selecting an existing measure, there are perhaps two that are most important: conceptual coherence with the study at hand and the quality and applicability of available validity and reliability evidence. First, *conceptual coherence* refers to the extent to which an existing instrument or scale measures the construct of interest in the study at hand. This term is not to be confused with an instrument's *validity,* which is defined as the extent to which an instrument measures what it purports to measure, but rather on the alignment between what the researcher seeks to measure and what the instrument was designed to measure. Novice researchers often make the mistake of selecting a measure that has *nominal coherence* with the construct they intent to study, but as the term implies, the alignment is in name only. As an example, *critical thinking* is defined in innumerable ways across disciplines. In some cases, critical thinking may be defined in a very domain-specific way, addressing only a limited range of narrow thinking and reasoning skills. In other instances, critical thinking may be defined as a general set of cognitive skills that are not bound to or restricted by a discipline or field of study. Clearly, using an instrument with items based on a narrow definition of critical thinking to measure broad critical thinking skills—often without an awareness of the distinction—could have profound consequences for the validity of study outcomes.

The second point to consider in selecting an instrument is the *quality and applicability of the available validity and reliability evidence.* Although I wish it were not so, too often, active instrument development and revision ceases after the publication of the initial psychometric paper detailing the development process and initial validity and reliability evidence. Because validity and reliability are not static concepts established once and for all by publication of a single-instrument development paper (Ironside & Spurlock, 2014), relying only on the initial development paper to support ongoing claims of robust validity and reliability can be a serious methodological mistake. From a practical perspective, it is exceedingly difficult to conduct all of the investigations at one time that are needed to support a broad range of validity claims. Supposing that one could do so, it would be an immense task to report these investigations with any level of detail in a single paper.

The same can be said of evidence for reliability. *Reliability,* by definition, is a concept that is time- and study subject bound. A Cronbach's alpha of .88 on a measure administered to a sample of 60 subjects, while an encouraging result for that single administration, is just a point estimate derived from the unique responses of a single group of subjects. Although we can have some confidence that reliability estimates will be sufficiently high when measures are taken in other similar populations, there is no guarantee of this, necessitating the need for continual testing and reporting of reliability metrics in published papers. Researchers considering an instrument for use in a study are well advised to evaluate multiple published assessments of reliability for a given measure and to give special attention to those reported by independent researchers and teams not affiliated with the instrument's initial development. If such evidence does not exist, as is commonly the case, in addition to exercising caution in selecting and using the measure, the researcher should consider this a possible limitation to the research.

KEY CONSIDERATIONS SUPPORTING A ROBUST SCIENCE OF NURSING EDUCATION

In the final section of this chapter, several key measurement-related considerations in support of building a robust science of nursing education are presented. These considerations are by no means an exhaustive list, but rather they reflect themes and issues identified and written about by others or are pervasive and persistent challenges discussed among nursing education researchers at national conference meetings, in editorial board meetings, and on research grant review panels. They are presented in no specific order.

Use Theoretically Appropriate and Empirically Sound Measures

As any experienced researcher can confirm, the conceptualization and planning phases of a research project are often the most time- and resource-intensive part of the research process—but also the most important. Locating, evaluating, and selecting measures is worth the time and effort in every case. The most appropriate instrument for a given study may not be the most popular instrument in use at the present time. A careful examination of validity and reliability evidence for a given measure may show that it performs reliably among one ethnic or racial group but not among others. Why? Perhaps researchers in other disciplines have seriously questioned a tool commonly used by nurse researchers. Are these concerns valid and relevant? It may be that a measure of health beliefs developed for administration to social workers can easily be used in a study of nurses, but the argument and data supporting this choice must be presented so that readers and reviewers can evaluate the question for themselves. In sum, taking the time to ensure that the measures selected for use in a study are theoretically sound and have a sufficient empirical basis is one of the most important steps a researcher can take to support trustworthy and generalizable study findings and conclusions.

Use Direct, Objective Measures Whenever Possible

Nursing education researchers must avoid making the mistake of equating the quality and accuracy of data collected via a direct, objective measure with data collected using a proxy measure. The term *proxy measure* is used to describe a substitute measure used when the measure of first choice is unavailable, is costly to procure, is more time consuming to administer, or was not designed for the method of administration the researcher desires (e.g., with measures designed to be administered in person instead of via online survey software). Proxy measures are not automatically *equivalent* to the measure for which they are substituting. Oftentimes they are thought to be *good enough,* but significant evidence suggests that this may be a poor assumption.

As noted previously, measures based on self-report almost always provide biased measurements that deviate far from measurements taken using more direct, objective methods (e.g., Zell & Krizan, 2014). Given the choice, why would a nursing education researcher rely on a student's self-reported skill level in providing health education to patients when direct observation of skill performance is possible? Perhaps this is due to limited funding for research staff to conduct the more time-intensive measurements, but more often it is for the sake of convenience and expediency. We must ask ourselves this question, however: Should research findings based on error-prone measurements be used to draw rational conclusions about the constructs of interest? If we answer honestly—no—we are forced then to consider that a different approach is needed, one where the discipline commits itself and its resources to developing sound measures that can be used by researchers committed to conducting rigorous research that will serve as the basis of evidence-based nursing education practice.

A related concern that bears mentioning here is similar in effect to using proxy measures (when more objective measures are available) but is much less obviously problematic. It involves identifying—perhaps misidentifying—antecedent, related, or proxy constructs as *outcomes* when they would be more correctly thought of as *processes.* Those familiar with advanced regression and modeling techniques may prefer the term *moderator* to describe these constructs; they are important variables to consider, but they are best conceptualized as predictors—not outcomes. An example of this is with the concept of self-efficacy.

As a concept, self-efficacy has a long history and a robust research base to support its importance and relevance to understanding and predicting human behavior. Simply put, *self-efficacy* is one's belief or confidence in his or her ability to carry out (or execute) certain behaviors or actions (Bandura, 1977). It is generally regarded as a motivational factor, consistently found to be correlated with a wide range of human behavior. It is not, however, a perfect predictor of behavior. In a recent meta-analysis examining the relationship between self-efficacy and behavioral performance, Sitzmann and Yeo (2013) found that whereas the overall correlation between self-efficacy beliefs and performance is moderate ($\rho = .42$, $k = 38$, $N = 5,414$), when moderating factors are considered, the effect of self-efficacy on performance is low or zero. Stizmann and Yeo report much stronger evidence for an effect of past performance on self-efficacy, suggesting that "self-efficacy is primarily a product of past performance rather than a driver of subsequent performance" (p. 558). Thus, treating self-efficacy as an outcome variable based on the assumption that it is a sufficient proxy for actual performance is deeply questionable. By way of example, if a researcher is interested in the effect of an interprofessional simulation training program on the conflict resolution skills of nursing students, the measurement strategy may include a conflict resolution self-efficacy measure, but this should be in addition to—not in lieu of—an actual demonstration of conflict resolution skills by the study subjects. Given the difficulty of identifying and studying even just the most important moderating variables influencing the relationship between self-efficacy and behavioral performance, the critical importance of directly measuring the outcome of most interest—to the greatest extent possible—cannot be understated.

Developing New Measures, Scales, and Instruments Is Fundamental to Advancing the Science of Nursing Education

A simple, seemingly self-evident fact is that if instrument or scale development were easy, this chapter would read very differently than it does—and may even be unnecessary in the first place. Developing new scales, measures, and instruments is time consuming, resource intensive, and too often underrewarded in academic nursing. DeVellis (2012) outlines the following general steps in the instrument development process: (a) determining clearly the construct to be measured, (b) generating the pool of scale items, (c) determining the format of the scale, (d) enlisting experts to review the candidate items, (e) considering the inclusion of validation items, (f) pilot administration of items, (g) evaluation and analysis of the pilot data, and (h) optimizing the length of the scale. Included within each of these steps is a multitude of steps and considerations that require different and sometimes, such as in the case of factor analysis of scale data, very technical expertise. Research-oriented doctoral programs in nursing and education—those most frequently attended by nurses—often provide insufficient education and training in instrument development, further limiting the capacity of future nursing education researchers to carry out this important work.

By design, master's and doctor of nursing practice programs provide even less exposure to the techniques, methods, and skills needed for instrument development. Thus, nursing education researchers interested in developing new instruments may need to obtain additional training and education in support of this goal. There are several existing options for this type of training. Examples include a nursing-oriented short summer course offered by the University of North Carolina at Chapel Hill School of Nursing (http://nursing.unc.edu/lifelong/summer-institutes-course-schedules/) and the survey-focused summer short courses offered by the Survey Research Center of the University of Michigan (http://si.isr.umich.edu/courses). The National League for Nursing (http://nln.org) also provides professional development opportunities through preconference instrument development workshops and a variety of conference sessions and publications focused on skill development in measurement and assessment. Researchers interested in accessible guidance on instrument or scale development are encouraged to review the widely cited work by DeVellis (2012); the newly released but very comprehensive health-focused text by Polit and Yang (2016); and the measurement text by Waltz, Strickland, and Lenz (2010), now in its fourth edition. Researchers interested in developing knowledge tests may refer to Thorndike and Thorndike-Christ

(2011) or Downing and Haladyna (2006), both classic works in the fields of education and psychology.

Another approach more immediately available to nursing education researchers is to collaborate with others who can bring the necessary skills to an instrument development project. This can take the form of local collaborations across departments and disciplines within a single college or university, or it could involve remote collaboration with team members more geographically separated. With available online collaboration technologies, it has never been easier to work effectively across distance, time zones, and organizational boundaries. Depending on the project, the members needed minimally include (a) a content/theory expert who can provide guidance on the nature of the construct to be measured and the intended use of the measure, and who can identify others, such as subject matter experts, to participate as needed in the instrument development process, and (b) a measurement/psychometrics expert who can provide guidance on the form the measure could take, item construction and generation, research design for initial testing, and statistical analysis support. In some cases, more than one person may share each of these roles.

An example "lean team" scenario is where a nursing education researcher serves as the content/theory expert, and a faculty collaborator with a background in educational psychology (frequently housed in departments or colleges of education), psychology, or statistics provides psychometric and data analysis support. As with any group effort where a scholarly product (e.g., a paper, book chapter, oral presentation) is produced, establishing clear role expectations and agreements on authorship early on is important for team cohesion and for avoiding conflicts later in the process. Instrument development teams may also need to work out issues of copyright ownership (of the resulting instrument) and whether members contributing to the project are viewed as consultants or full members of the research team who contribute to and take responsibility for the whole project.

CONCLUSIONS AND IMPLICATIONS

In a stark statement illustrating the fundamental importance of measurement to the research process, DeVellis (2012) wrote, "A researcher who does not understand the relationship between measures and the variables they represent, in a very literal sense, does not know what they are talking about. Viewed in this light, the efforts entailed in careful measurement are amply rewarded by their benefits" (p. 191). As noted, and please forgive my insistence on restating this, it is impossible to address all of the substantive measurement issues germane to nursing education research in just one chapter, or even in a whole volume. In highlighting some of the most important ones, however, it is my hope that these considerations make their way into the deliberations that shape the future of the science of nursing education, both at the local research project planning level and nationally, in professional and leadership circles. As DeVellis so aptly stated, errors or omissions in measurement can have make-or-break consequences for a study. When accumulated over time and throughout the evidence base for a discipline, the consequences are magnified, undermining the discipline's effectiveness—and ultimately its impact and contributions—to the society it serves.

References

Artino, A. R., La Rochelle, J. S., Dezee, K. J., & Gehlbach, H. (2014). Developing question-naires for educational research: AMEE Guide No. 87. *Medical Teacher, 36*, 463–474. doi:10.3109/0142159X.2014.889814

Bandura, A. (1977). Self-efficacy: Toward a unifying theory of behavioral change. *Psychological Review, 84*, 191–215. doi:10.1037/0033-295X.84.2.191

Barry, A. E., Chaney, B. H., Piazza-Gardner, A. K., & Chavarria, E. A. (2014). Validity and reliability reporting practices in the field of health education and behavior: A review of seven journals. *Health Education and Behavior, 41*, 12–18. doi:10.1177/1090198113483139

Barry, A. E., Chaney, E. H., Stellefson, M. L., & Chaney, J. D. (2011). So you want to develop a survey: Practical recommenda-tions for scale development. *American Journal of Health Studies, 26*, 97–105.

Bowman, N. A. (2010). Can 1st-year college students accurately report their learn-ing and development?. *American Edu-cational Research Journal, 47*, 466–496. doi:10.3102/0002831209353595

Carlson, J. F., Geisinger, K. F., & Jonson, J. L. (Eds.). (2014). *The nineteenth mental measure-ments yearbook*. Lincoln, NE: Buros Center for Testing.

Chinn, P. L., & Kramer, M. K. (2014). *Theory and nursing: Integrated knowledge development in nursing* (9th ed.). St. Louis, MO: Mosby.

De Champlain, A. F. (2010). A primer on classi-cal test theory and item response theory for assessments in medical education. *Medical Education, 44*, 109–117. doi:10.1111/j.13652923.2009.03425.x

DeVellis, R. F. (2012). *Scale development: Theory and applications* (3rd ed.). Los Angeles: Sage.

Downing, S. M. (2003). Item response theory: Applications of modern test theory in medi-cal education. *Medical Education, 37*, 739–745. doi:10.1046/j.1365-2923.2003.01587.x

Downing, S. M., & Haladyna, T. M. (2006). *Handbook of test development*. Mahwah, NJ: L. Erlbaum.

Dunning, D., & Helzer, E. G. (2014). Beyond the correlation coefficient in studies of self-assessment accuracy commentary on Zell & Krizan (2014). *Perspectives on Psychological Science, 9*, 126–130. doi:10.1177/1745691614521244

Educational Testing Service, Inc. (2015). *ETS Test Link Database*. Princeton, NJ. Retrieved from https://www.ets.org/test_link/about

Insight Assessment, Inc. (2016). California Critical Thinking Skills Test. San Jose, CA: Author.

Ironside, P. M., & Spurlock, D. R. (2014). Get-ting serious about building nursing educa-tion science. *Journal of Nursing Education, 53*, 667–669. doi:10.3928/01484834-20141118-10

Kottner, J., Audigé, L., Brorson, S., Donner, A., Gajewski, B. J., Hróbjartsson, A., et al. (2011). Guidelines for Reporting Reliability and Agreement Studies (GRRAS) were pro-posed. *Journal of Clinical Epidemiology, 64*, 96–106. doi:10.1016/j.jclinepi.2010.03.002

Lucas, N. P., Macaskill, P., Irwig, L., & Bogduk, N. (2010). The development of a qual-ity appraisal tool for studies of diagnostic reliability (QAREL). *Journal of Clinical Epidemiology, 63*, 854–861. doi:10.1016/j.jclinepi.2009.10.002

Martin, J., Sugarman, J., & Slaney, K. (Eds.). (2015). *The Wiley handbook of theoretical and philosophical psychology: Methods, approaches, and new directions for social sciences*. Malden, MA: Wiley-Blackwell.

McDonald, M. (2014). *The nurse educator's guide to assessing learning outcomes*. Burlington, MA: Jones & Bartlett Learning.

McEwen, M., & Wills, E. M. (2014). *Theoretical basis for nursing* (4th ed.). Philadelphia: Lippincott Williams & Wilkins.

Patient Reported Outcome Measurement Information System. (2013). *PROMIS® Instrument Development and Validation Scientific Standards Version 2.0 (revised May 2013)*. Retrieved June 9, 2016, from http://www.nihpromis.org/Documents/PROMISStandards_Vers2.0_Final.pdf

Pittenger, D. J. (2005). Cautionary comments regarding the Myers-Briggs Type Indicator. *Consulting Psychology Journal: Practice and Research, 57*, 210–221. doi:10.1037/1065-9293.57.3.210

Polit, D. F., & Yang, F. (2016). *Measurement and the measurement of change: A primer for the health professions*. Philadelphia: Wolters Kluwer/Lippincott Williams & Wilkins.

Sijtsma, K. (2009). On the use, the misuse, and the very limited usefulness of Cronbach's alpha. *Psychometrika, 74*, 107–120. doi:10.1007/s11336-008-9101-0

Sitzmann, T., & Yeo, G. (2013). A meta-analytic investigation of the within-person self-efficacy domain: Is self-efficacy a product of past performance or a driver of future performance? *Personnel Psychology, 66*, 531–568. doi:10.1111/peps.12035

Spurlock, D., & Wonder, A. H. (2015). Validity and reliability evidence for a new measure: The evidence-based practice knowledge assessment in nursing. *Journal of Nursing Education, 54*, 605–613. doi:10.3928/01484834-20151016-01

Streiner, D. L., & Kottner, J. (2014). Recommendations for reporting the results of studies of instrument and scale development and testing. *Journal of Advanced Nursing, 70*, 1970–1979. doi:10.1111/jan.12402

Thorndike, R. M., & Thorndike-Christ, T. M. (2011). *Measurement and evaluation in psychology and education* (8th ed.). Boston: Pearson.

Waltz, C., Strickland, O. L., & Lenz, E. (Eds.). (2010). *Measurement in nursing and health research* (4th ed.). New York: Springer.

Zell, E., & Krizan, Z. (2014). Do people have insight into their abilities? A metasynthesis. *Perspectives on Psychological Science, 9*, 111–125. doi:10.1177/1745691613518075

5

Design-Based Educational Research in Nursing

Anne M. Krouse, PhD, MBA, RN-BC

The National League for Nursing (NLN) (2012), in *NLN Vision: Transforming Research in Nursing Education,* called for "building linkages between practice and education; advancing the science of nursing education through the development of more rigorous and robust research designs and evaluation protocols" (p. 1). Pedagogical research in nursing education has done little to build the science in ways that can be applied, replicated, and built upon. There are numerous examples of nursing education interventions that have been examined, including case studies, problem-based learning, and concept maps. What is lacking in the literature is attention to the design in the development and discussion of the educational intervention.

Why is design in the development of an educational intervention so important? The design is the "how to" of the intervention. It is the steps that produce the outcome. To test the reliability of a design with other samples of students, the steps must be clearly articulated so that they can be replicated. In doing so, the effectiveness of the design in relation to the desired outcome measures can be empirically tested. Purposeful refinement of the design can also serve as an opportunity to improve outcomes by providing evidence to support those changes. It is this cyclic nature of design testing that allows for the development of evidence-based educational interventions. According to McKenney and Reeves (2012):

> Sustainable use of new ideas does not come when an intervention focuses on using new resources or changing overt behaviors. Real change can come when we focus not only on what and how things can be done, but when we also work to understand *why.* (pp. 1–2)

Similarly, although theoretical support for the educational intervention study may be implicit in the research design, there is often a lack of theoretical underpinnings for the development of the intervention itself. Theory is used in the design of the empirical study to identify concepts and constructs that will be measured; however, theory also needs to be considered in the design of the intervention to inform the design. In that way, the findings of the empirical study advance both theories. This type of educational research, referred to as design-based research, is used to provide theoretical evidence both *through* the use of educational interventions as well as *on* the intervention itself (Cobb, Confrey, diSessa, Lehrer, & Schaulbe, 2003; McKenney & Reeves, 2012).

The purpose of this chapter is to provide an overview of design-based educational research and its application to the science of nursing education.

DESIGN-BASED EDUCATIONAL RESEARCH

"What sets educational design research apart from other forms of scientific inquiry is its commitment to developing theoretical insights and practical solutions simultaneously in real world contexts together with the stakeholders" (McKenney & Reeves, 2012, p. 7). Educational research is context dependent, and to ignore the context in the design of the study limits the strength of the evidence attributed to the intervention. What is needed in research is to identify those contextual variables that may affect the outcomes of the intervention and empirically test and refine them through iterative testing of the intervention. "Educational design research is structured to explore, rather than mute, the complex realities of teach and learning contexts and respond accordingly" (McKenney & Reeves, 2012, p. 15).

Design-based educational research is "a genre of research in which the iterative development of solutions to practical and complex educational problems also provides the context for empirical investigation, which yields theoretical understanding that can inform the work of others" (McKenney & Reeves, 2012, p. 7). It has been referred to by several terms, including *design-based research, development research, design experiments, formative research,* and *educational design research* (McKenney & Reeves, 2012).

The purposes of design-based research are to test a theory and to design and refine the intervention. Although both purposes exist, one purpose may initially drive the research (McKenney & Reeves, 2012). The intervention may be the means for testing specific constructs and concepts of a theory guiding the empirical design of the study. The concepts and constructs are related to, but not necessarily the same as, the intervention itself. This type of design-based research is called *research "through" interventions.* In *research "on" interventions,* the primary purpose is studying the characteristics of the intervention and the relative conditions related to the implementation of the intervention (McKenney & Reeves, 2012). Both purposes contribute to advancing theoretical understanding. Additionally, the refinement of the intervention through empirical testing provides evidence to support teaching practices. According to Abdallah and Wergerif (2014):

> Unlike experimental research, DBR does not target the mere implementation of theories, designs, and models in a controlled fashion. Rather, it seeks to improve both theory and the educational context itself which is seen as a messy reality that should be studied as it is. (pp. 3–4)

Nieveen, McKenney, and van den Akker (2006) delineated the types of design studies in terms of process: validation, development, and effectiveness. A validation study is one where the testing and generation of theory is the goal. Those theories guide development studies where the desired outcome is the production of an intervention and design theory relative to that intervention. Finally, the effectiveness of the intervention must be tested in a variety of contexts. According to Herrington and Reeves (2011):

> At every stage of the research process, initial and evolving design principles inform and guide the direction and shape of innovation being developed as well as its implementation and testing, until ultimately, the evolution of draft guidelines into refined design principles become a critical product of the research. (p. 596)

The Design-Based Research Collective (DRC), a group of researchers committed to advancing this type of research, suggested five characteristics that should be present for good design-based research. The first characteristic is that the goals of theory development and design are intertwined. Second, "cycles of design, enactment, analysis, and redesign" are the core of development and research (Design-Based Research Collective [DRC], 2003, p. 5). The third characteristic is related to the output of the research in that it must lead to the dissemination of theories that communicate implications to those in practice. An account of how the design functions in "authentic settings" in relation to the contextual issues is the fourth characteristic. Finally, "the development of such accounts relies on methods that can document and connect processes of enactment to outcomes of interest" (DRC, 2003, p. 5). The potential benefits of design-based research include the creation of novel teaching and learning environments, the development of contextually based theories of learning, the advancement of design knowledge, and an increase in the capacity for educational innovation (DRC, 2003).

Instructional Design

Designing an educational intervention involves analyzing the problem, designing the process and procedure for the educational intervention, and the design solution (Edelson, 2002). "Instructional design is a field concerned with systematic processes for developing instruction to reliably yield desired learning and performance results" (McKenney & Reeves, 2012, p. 61). Theory is used in instructional design to describe the "how" and "why" of the design solution.

Instructional design has roots in behaviorism and general systems theory. Instructional design seeks to elicit a response from a learner (behaviorism) given a set of learning conditions. Using a systems approach, the goal of instructional design is responding to "multiple components that form the system, the interactions within a system, and the interactions that occur between different systems" (Branch & Merrill, 2012, p. 8).

There are several instructional design models; however, the ADDIE (Figure 5.1) paradigm represents the core elements of most instructional design models. The components of ADDIE are analysis, design, development, implementation, and evaluation (Branch & Merrill, 2012).

During the *analysis* phase, the problem is identified and learning goals are set. *Design* involves the development of measurable learning objectives, classification of the type of learning, and the specification of learning activities. *Development* of instructional materials follows in preparation for *implementation* of the design. Finally, formative and summative *evaluation* informs refinement of the design and measures the effectiveness of the intervention (Branch & Merrill, 2012).

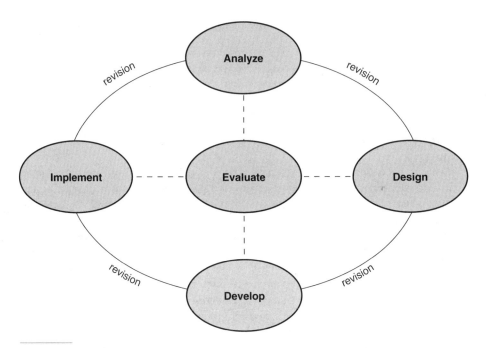

FIGURE 5.1 ADDIE Model of Instructional Design. (From *Survey of Instructional Development Models* [4th ed.] by K. L. Gustafson and R. M. Branch, 2002, p. 3. Public Domain, 2002, ERIC Clearinghouse on Information & Technology.)

Generic Model for Design Research in Education

McKenney and Reeves (2012) outlined a generic model for design-based research in education involving three iterative, flexible phases: *analysis, design,* and *evaluation.* Inherent in the model is a dual focus on theory and practice, integrated research and design processes, and theoretical and practical outcomes (McKenney & Reeves, 2012).

Analysis

The first step in the process is defining and analyzing the problem. A holistic approach to the analysis should be taken, using a root cause analysis methodology to identify those aspects of the problem that will become the target of the intervention. Equally important in the analysis is to identify the contextual factors that may affect the design of the intervention (McKenney & Reeves, 2012). The contextual factors may or may not be able to be controlled in the design, but their potential influence on the design, as well as the outcomes of the intervention, should be carefully considered. A literature review is used to explore the elements of the problems, empirically based data about the problem, and theoretical connections that may inform the design. Exploring problems that are similar, along with the targeted solutions, is the next step. The expected outcome of this phase is the clear articulation of the problem, beginning design requirements and propositions, and the emergence of a theoretical connection (McKenney & Reeves, 2012).

Design

The design process involves the delineation of design requirements, design propositions, and a theoretical framework to guide the design. Design requirements are the criteria needed to meet the learning goals and the conditions under which the design will be implemented (McKenney & Reeves, 2012). The design propositions delineate the specifics of what the design will look like, including how and why it will be developed that way. The theoretical framework informs the requirements and propositions. Congruence of the theory with the design ensures treatment validity of the study (Hoadley, 2004).

To make the intervention able to be replicated, it should be clear, value added, compatible, and tolerant. A clear design is one that can easily be followed and makes sense to the educator using that design. To be able to use the design, educators must perceive that there is additional value to its use. Additionally, educators will use designs that reflect their beliefs, culture, and practices. "Tolerance refers to how precisely core components must be enacted if the intervention to be true to its goals" (McKenney & Reeves, 2012, p. 166). It is expected that the design will undergo some variability in its implementation due to the influence of the contexts within the learning environment. Some flexibility should be built into the design to improve its tolerance.

Evaluation and Reflection

Because of the dual nature of the purposes of design-based research, the evaluation process may include an evaluation of the outcomes of the intervention in relation to the theory guiding the study and/or may evaluate the design of the intervention itself in relation to the theory informing the design, or quite possibly both. Areas of evaluation may include soundness, viability, effectiveness, impact, and usefulness in other contexts. Theoretical understanding comes from reflection on the empirical findings. The knowledge generated from the study may inform the intervention design, the theoretical support for that design, and/or the theory guiding the empirical study in relation to the concepts or constructs represented by the intervention (McKenney & Reeves, 2012).

WHY IS DESIGN IMPORTANT IN NURSING EDUCATION RESEARCH?

Advancing the science of nursing education requires strong evidence that supports curricular development and robust educational practices that result in the achievement of student learning goals. Much of the research in nursing education reported that focuses on the effectiveness of educational interventions has not clearly tied the effectiveness of that intervention to the design of the intervention, thus limiting the usefulness of that intervention in other contexts. Without clarity with regard to design, there is little likelihood of replication and subsequent testing and refinement of that intervention. Additionally, the validity of the intervention itself comes into question when the research on the intervention in conducted at a single site with a single sample of learners and implemented by a single teacher. Research that focuses only on outcomes has little relationship to the design of the intervention (McKenney & Reeves, 2012).

Emerson and Records (2008) defined evidence-based teaching practices as the incorporation of the *doing* of the teaching with the *study* of the teaching. Unfortunately, there is a lack of evidence supporting the effectiveness of curricular design and teaching innovations in nursing education research (Ferguson & Day, 2005). In a study of faculty perspectives on evidence-based teaching practices in nursing education, participants rated the availability of sufficient evidence to make changes in nursing education the lowest ($M = 3.05$), with qualitative comments about lack of quality evidence needed to identify and enact changes in nursing education (Kalb, O'Connor-Von, Brockway, Rierson, & Sendelbach, 2015).

To build the science of nursing education, Broome, Ironside, and McNelis (2012) call for not only knowledge generation but also "continual testing and refinement by those who apply the knowledge" (p. 524). Incorporating design in educational intervention research will provide the means to iteratively test the efficacy of those interventions in different contexts. Similarly, Diekelmann (2005) emphasized the importance of studying issues over time. Single-site, one-time testing of an educational intervention does little to determine the reliability of the effectiveness of that intervention, particularly if the design of that intervention has not been given rigorous consideration and delineation in publications/presentations arising from that research. Ironside and Spurlock (2014) state that "when disseminated, these studies rarely have the control, power, comparison groups, or methodological sophistication required for generalizability. This limits the application of findings outside of the study site and does little to build nursing education science" (p. 668).

Attention to the design of the intervention in nursing education research would move the science forward. A well-designed educational intervention can be subjected to testing and refinement in multiple learning contexts over time. Measurable outcomes that are directly related to the design can be evaluated to determine the effectiveness of the intervention. Ultimately, this can lead to a robust level of evidence contributing to the science of nursing education, which can be translated into practice.

Nurse Faculty Use of Instructional Design

An issue to be considered is nurse faculty readiness to design theoretically supported educational interventions. Gross (2006) investigated experienced nurse faculty's use of instructional design in their teaching processes and found that although none of the six participants had any training or stated that they used instructional design in the conduct of their courses, they all exhibited behaviors reflecting the ADDIE steps in their teaching. Similarly, Elkind (2009) studied nurse faculty's training and competency in instructional design in schools of nursing that offered online nursing programs. She found that they lacked instructional design training and that the programs she investigated did not provide training or support related to instructional design for faculty teaching in online courses.

Collaboration with instructional designers may be a consideration in the development of a well-designed educational intervention. The instructional designer can provide expertise in creating a systematic design in response to an identified learning problem. Additionally, nursing master's and doctoral programs focused on nursing education should include a focus on design in their discussions of evidence-based teaching practice. The generic educational research design process should be an area of development for all nursing education investigators.

EXAMPLES OF DESIGN-BASED NURSING EDUCATION RESEARCH

Nursing education research examples with a focus on intervention design primarily are found in the areas of simulation and online education. The studies vary in their rigor, level of development of the design, and connection to theory. The explicit articulation of the design as an educational intervention is seen in all of the following studies.

Design and Simulation

One of the best examples of the use of design in nursing simulation literature is the Jeffries (2016) simulation framework, later renamed the *NLN/Jeffries simulation framework* (NLN/JSF). The model has five components with associated variables: teacher, student, educational practices, design and characteristics of simulation (intervention), and outcomes. The areas of design of the simulation are objectives, planning, fidelity, complexity, cues, and debriefing. Jeffries states that an empirically based and consistent framework is needed to assess outcomes of simulations and to conduct research in this area in a systematic manner.

As part of an NLN project team, Groom, Henderson, and Sitner (2014) examined the literature to determine the state of the science regarding the NLN/JSF on the characteristics of the simulation design construct. There are five key subcomponents of this construct: objectives, fidelity, problem solving, student support, and debriefing. The authors found that terminology was a significant issue in their review of the literature. The NLN/JSF was not consistently noted in the literature review; however, similar educational practices on which the design is based were noted throughout the literature. They suggested that the use and standardization of reporting on simulations in this format would lead to better reproducibility and called for future research to focus on the impact of the simulation design characteristics on "learning outcomes, learning transfer, duration of effect, and translational impacts" (Groom, Henderson, & Sitner, 2014, p. 343).

Taking a different approach, Chmil, Turk, Adamson, and Larew (2015) developed a new experiential learning simulation design incorporating principles of active learning using the experiential learning theory of Kolb (1984). An experimental group of first-semester prelicensure baccalaureate nursing students ($n = 72$) completed the simulation with structured briefing activities, whereas the control group ($n = 72$) used independent briefing activities. The same procedures and faculty were used for both groups for the performing and debriefing phases of the simulation. The simulation design used for the control group was the nursing education simulation framework (Jeffries, 2005). Clinical judgment was measured using the Lasater (2007) clinical judgment rubric (LCJR), and the simulation behaviors were measured using the Creighton Simulation Evaluation Instrument (CSE-I®) (www.nursing.creighton.edu). The mean of the LCJR was significantly higher in the experimental group ($M = 27.81$, $p < .01$) than the control group ($M = 20.75$). There was a statistically significant relationship among the scores of the LCJR and the CSE-I for the experimental group ($r = .069$, $p < .01$). The authors concluded that the experiential learning simulation design was more effective than the nursing education simulation framework.

Design and Online Nursing Education

Jeffries (2005) used the hyperlearning model originally published by the same author in 2000 (Jeffries, 2000) to develop an online critical care course. The model is based on principles for best practices in education of Chickering and Gamson (1987). Once the course was developed, two students and one web specialist reviewed the course for usability using a rubric designed by the evaluation team, examining course design, instructional design, and content. Following modifications that were made after the usability testing, pilot testing occurred with 15 senior baccalaureate nursing students and RNs. The instruments used included an investigator-designed knowledge test; a skills competence checklist; and the Evaluating Educational Uses of the Web in Nursing (EEUWIN) instrument (Billings, Connors, & Skiba, 2001), which measured student satisfaction, best practices in undergraduate education, and convenience. All students achieved a passing score on the knowledge test and completed the skills competence checklist. The means for all of the best practices were above the national benchmark (active learning, $M = 3.74$; prompt feedback, $M = 3.98$, student-faculty interaction, $M = 3.54$, diverse styles of learning, $M = 4.20$), with the exception of collaboration at $M = 2.63$ (national benchmark, $M = 3.01$). Students also reported a high level of satisfaction with the course ($M = 4.17$) and perceived a high level of convenience ($M = 4.01$).

Using a different design model, Harper (2007) examined student affective outcomes related to ageism in a quasiexperimental study. The Pebble-in-the-Pond model of instructional design by Merrill (2002) was used to design an online gerontology nursing course. Eight students participated in the experimental group, and eight students participated in the control group, which received the standard gerontology course. Harper (2007) found that affective learning, as evidenced by decreased ageism, was found in the experimental group but not in the control group. Although this was a single-site, small sample study, it is a good example of how design can be connected to student outcomes.

Holtslander, Racine, Furniss, Burles, and Turner (2012) used the 4C/ID model by van Merriënboer, Bastiaens, and Hoogveld (2004), a holistic instructional design model used for complex learning tasks that require the learner to apply skills in the real world, to develop an online course to teach qualitative research methods to a group of interdisciplinary graduate students ($N = 17$) (nursing, psychology, medicine, and sociology). The theory underlying the design was constructivism. The steps of the 4C/ID model are: tasks should be authentic and whole task in nature, provide students with support information, provide students information just at the time they need it, and allow opportunities for part-task performance. The investigators used course evaluations to measure the success of the design stating that the students felt the course design was effective and that they established a good learning community in the class. The lack of rigorous empirical outcome data was a weakness of the study; however, the discussion of the analysis and design process met the criteria for design-based research.

CONCLUSIONS AND IMPLICATIONS

Advancing the science of nursing education is going to require the development of evidence-based teaching practices. Research through and on educational interventions must be part of that evidence. Attention to theoretically based, well-constructed, and articulated intervention designs within an empirical study will allow for replication, refinement, and further testing of that intervention. Graduate programs in nursing education must foster student knowledge development in the educational design process. The results of well-designed intervention research will yield new educational theories, new knowledge regarding existing theories, evidence-based effective educational interventions, and emerging design principles.

References

Abdallah, M. S., & Wegerif, R. B. (2014). Design-based research (DBR) in educational enquiry and technological studies: A version for PhD students targeting the integration of new technologies and literacies into educational contexts. *ERIC*. Retrieved June 9, 2016, from http://eric.ed.gov/?id=ED546471

Billings, D., Connors, H., & Skiba, D. (2001). Benchmarking best practices in web-based nursing courses. *Advances in Nursing Science, 23*(3), 41–52. doi:10.1097/00012272-200103000-00005

Branch, R., & Merrill, M. D. (2012) Characteristics of instructional design models. In R. Resiser, & J. Dempsey (Eds.), *Trends and issues in instructional design and technology* (3rd ed., pp. 8–16). Boston: Pearson.

Broome, M. E., Ironside, P. M., & McNelis, A. M. (2012). Research in nursing education: State of the science. *Journal of Nursing Education, 51*, 521–524. doi: 10.3928/01484834-20120820-10

Chickering, A., & Gamson, Z. (1987). Seven principles of good practice in undergraduate education. *American Association for Higher Education Bulletin, 39*(7), 3–7. doi:10.1016/0307-4412(89)90094-0

Chmil, J. V., Turk, M., Adamson, K., & Larew, C. (2015). Effects of an experiential learning simulation design on clinical nursing judgment development. *Nurse Educator, 40*, 228–232. doi:10.1097/NNE.0000000000000159

Cobb, P., Confrey, J., diSessa, A., Lehrer, R., & Schauble, L. (2003). Design experiments in educational research. *Educational Researcher, 32*(1), 9–13. doi:10.3102/0013189x032001009

Design-Based Research Collective. (2003). Design-based research: An emerging paradigm for educational inquiry. *Educational Researcher, 32*(1), 5–8. doi:10.3102/0013189x032001005

Diekelmann, N. (2005). Creating an inclusive science for nursing education. *Nursing Education Perspectives, 26*, 64–65.

Edelson, D. C. (2002). Design research: What we learn when we engage in design. *Journal of the Learning Sciences, 11*(1), 105–121. doi:10.1207/s15327809jls1101_4

Elkind, E. C. (2009). *Nursing faculty's training in instructional design for online course development*. Unpublished doctoral dissertation. Retrieved from Proquest Central (Order No. 3315956).

Emerson, R. J., & Records, K. (2008). Today's challenge, tomorrow's excellence: The practice of evidence-based education. *Journal of Nursing Education, 47*, 359–370. doi:10.3928/01484834-20080801-04

Ferguson, L., & Day, R. (2005). Evidence-based nursing education: Myth or reality? *Journal of Nursing Education, 44*, 107–115.

Groom, J. A., Henderson, D., & Sittner, B. J. (2014). NLN/Jeffries simulation framework state of the science project: Simulation design characteristics. *Clinical Simulation in Nursing, 10*, 337–344. doi:10.1016/j.ecns.2013.02.004

Gross, M. D. (2006). *Instructional design thought processes of expert nurse educators*. Unpublished doctoral dissertation. Retrieved from Proquest Central (Order No. 3278698).

Harper, S. P. (2007). *Instructional design for affective learning in online nursing education*. Unpublished doctoral dissertation. Retrieved from ProQuest Central (Order No. 3246873).

Herrington, J., & Reeves, T. C. (2011). Using design principles to improve pedagogical practice and promote student engagement. Proceedings from Ascilite 2011: *Changing Demands, Changing Directions*. Retrieved June 9, 2016, from http://www.ascilite.org/conferences/hobart11/downloads/papers/Herrington-full.pdf

Hoadley, C. (2004). Methodological alignment in design-based research. *Educational Psychologist, 39*, 203–212. doi:10.1207/s15326985ep3904_2

Holtslander, L. F., Racine, L., Furniss, S., Burles, M., & Turner, H. (2012). Developing and piloting an online graduate nursing course focused on experiential learning of qualitative research methods. *Journal of Nursing Education, 51*, 345–348. doi:10.3928/01484834-20120427-03

Ironside, P. M., & Spurlock, D. J. (2014). Getting serious about building nursing education science. *Journal of Nursing Education, 53*, 667–669. doi:10.3928/01484834-20141118-10

Jeffries, P. (2000). Development and test of a model for designing interactive CD ROMs for teaching nursing skills. *Computers in Nursing, 18*, 118–124.

Jeffries, P. (2005). Development and testing of a hyperlearning model for design of an online critical care course. *Journal of Nursing Education, 44*, 366–372.

Jeffries, P. R. (2016). *The NLN Jeffries Simulation Theory*. Philadelphia: Wolters Kluwer/National League for Nursing.

Kalb, K. A., O'Conner-Von, S. K., Brockway, C., Rierson, C. L., & Sendelbach, S. (2015). Evidence-based teaching practice in nursing education: Faculty perspectives and practices. *Nursing Education Perspectives, 36*, 212–219. doi:10.5480/14-1472

Kolb, D. A. (1984). *Experiential learning: Experience as the source of learning and development*. Upper Saddle River, NJ: Prentice Hall.

Lasater K. (2007). Clinical judgment development: Using simulation to create an assessment rubric. *Journal of Nursing Education, 46*, 496–503.

McKenney, S., & Reeves, T. C. (2012). *Conducting educational design research*. New York: Routledge.

Merrill, D. (2002). A Pebble-in-the-Pond model for instructional design. *Performance Improvement, 41*(7), 39–44. doi:10.1002/pfi.4140410709

National League for Nursing. (2012). *NLN Vision: Transforming research in nursing education: A living document from the National League for Nursing*. Retrieved June 9, 2016, from http://www.nln.org/docs/default-source/about/nln-vision-series-%28position-statements%29/nlnvision_5.pdf?sfvrsn=4

Nieveen, N., McKenney, S., & Van den Akker, J. (2006). Educational design research: The value of variety. In J. Van den Akker, K. Gravemeijer, S. McKenney, & N. Nieveen (Eds.). *Educational design research* (pp. 151–158). London: Routledge.

Van Merriënboer, J., Bastiaens, T., & Hoogveld, A. (2004). Instructional design for integrated e-learning. In W. Jochems, J. Van Merriënboer, & R. Koper (Eds.), *Integrated e-learning: Implications for pedagogy, technology and organization* (pp. 13–23). London: Routledge Falmer.

6

Ethical Inquiry in Research in Nursing Education

Barbara J. Patterson, PhD, RN, ANEF

Where is the evidence? Nurse faculty commonly raise this question when they are considering the implementation of changes in curricula, teaching strategies, assessment, or evaluation. Faculty can no longer teach the way they were taught; schools of nursing are being held accountable for student outcomes by accrediting bodies, students, and society. Ethically, as stewards of the discipline, faculty have a responsibility to contribute to professional knowledge (American Nurses Association, 2015), and conducting research is one of the critical elements of building the science of nursing education (Gresley, 2009). An evidence-based teaching practice is the gold standard and is contingent on studies that are rigorous and ethically conducted.

The body of research evidence in nursing education is growing, with more faculty conducting research on teaching and how students learn. Students are often recruited as research subjects by faculty and as student investigators for reasons of easy access, availability, time constraints, and limited funding, as well as professional scholarship obligations (Aycock & Currie, 2013; Comer, 2009; DuBois, 2002). Sometimes studies are designed with this population in mind. Nevertheless, students are in a dependent relationship with faculty, and as such their rights and welfare warrant safeguarding. Maintaining the integrity of the research process and minimizing the risk to research participants need to be at the forefront for all investigators.

This chapter focuses on the ethical conduct of research in the educational setting. There is a discussion of the challenges and key issues to consider when applying the principles of ethical conduct of research to students as participants. Strategies are presented that can be implemented before and during the research process to minimize participant risk.

THE NATURE OF EDUCATIONAL RESEARCH

Research is essential to the advancement of education. However, what constitutes research in the education setting and whether it warrants oversight by an institutional review board (IRB) has been a controversial subject for many years (DuBois, 2002). Questions arise as to whether the data are being used for curricular assessment or for research purposes. Teaching and learning is standard educational practice, with research being something more. Nevertheless, the distinction is not always clear, and ethically, the protection of students as research participants should always be the priority. DuBois (2002) emphasized this point by noting that "there is a conflict of interest inherent in educational research that could compromise student learning" (p. 4).

What is research? The Office for Human Research Protections (OHRP) defines *research* as "a systematic investigation, including research development, testing and evaluation, designed to develop or contribute to generalizable knowledge" (Code of Federal Regulations [CFR], 2009, p. 4). The primary intent of an activity often can assist an investigator in deciding whether or not the proposed activity is research. Is the investigator's primary intent to contribute to generalizable knowledge, whether through presentation or publication? Or will the data be used to implement changes in a single course? Unfortunately, there are times when this distinction is blurred in that "the data-gathering activity may itself be educational, the data may be used to improve the course in which students are participating, and the data may be used to further the science of education and the career of the investigator" (DuBois, 2002, p. 3). There is no guarantee of educational gain for the student. Teaching and learning should always take precedence over research to avoid any potential conflict of interest (Kirkwood, 2012).

To extend the OHRP's definition of research, the American Educational Research Association (AERA) elaborates for educators that education research encompasses

> the scientific field of study that examines education and learning processes and the human attributes, interactions, organizations, and institutions that shape educational outcomes. Scholarship in the field seeks to describe, understand, and explain how learning takes place throughout a person's life and how formal and informal contexts of education affect all forms of learning. Education research embraces the full spectrum of rigorous methods appropriate to the questions being asked and also drives the development of new tools and methods. (American Educational Research Association, 2015, para. 1).

Building the science of nursing education necessitates the use of rigorous methods to examine how nursing students learn and identify the best approaches to achieve optimal curricular outcomes. Developing reliable and valid instruments to capture assessment data and outcomes critical in the development of nursing students requires multiple phases of research with those who best inform the teaching-learning phenomena, specifically nursing students. All of these processes require ethical treatment of the participants.

ETHICAL RESEARCH: RESPECT, BENEFICENCE, AND JUSTICE

As defined by Resnik (2011), *ethics* are the "norms for conduct that distinguish between acceptable and unacceptable behavior (para. 1). . . . Ethical norms also serve the aims or goals of research and apply to people who conduct scientific research or other scholarly or creative activities" (para. 6). The *Belmont Report* (U.S. Department of Health and Human Services [HHS], 1979) established the ethical standards for research in the United States. The report identifies three basic principles relevant to the conduct of research with human subjects. These principles are respect, beneficence, and justice. They provide a framework to inform and guide investigators as they conceptualize and design their research studies. Each principle is discussed, and the application of the principles with respect to educational research and student participants is considered in a later section of the chapter.

The moral requirements for *respect for persons* include acknowledgement of autonomy and protection of those with limited autonomy (HHS, 1979). Autonomy involves the freedom of choice and implies voluntary informed consent that is not coerced. Those individuals who lack autonomy can be considered vulnerable. Whether college students as research participants are treated as a vulnerable population needs to be given due consideration. Nursing students have not traditionally been described as vulnerable, and most are likely to be capable of understanding the principle of autonomy (Clark & McCann, 2005); however, the dual nature of the student-teacher/participant-investigator relationship can generate a potential ethical conflict of interest (Anderson, 2011; Shi, 2006). Ferguson, Yonge, and Myrick (2004) framed this ethical conflict with the concept of double agency, or fulfilling two roles simultaneously, and they discussed its application to research conducted on one's students. It is incumbent on investigators to recognize double agency and design and to implement appropriate strategies to minimize risk and vulnerability with their students in the participant role.

Acknowledging that students are in a dependent relationship with faculty is a first step in safeguarding students' rights as research participants (Cleary, Walter, & Jackson, 2014). Power differentials exist in student-teacher relationships and can impact the students' right to opt out of research participation. Students may perceive this lack of autonomy and a sense of coercion since they are captive participants (Anderson, 2011). It is the fiduciary responsibility of faculty to facilitate learning with the "more powerful person entrusted to protect the best interests of the less powerful or dependent person" (Ferguson et al., 2004). Trust in these relationships is crucial in safeguarding the learning environment and conducting ethically sound research.

Beneficence is the second moral requirement highlighted in the *Belmont Report.* The report emphasizes the obligation of "do no harm" and to "maximize possible benefits and minimize possible harms" (HHS, 1979, para. 15). Protecting the well-being of all study participants and treating them with respect is a crucial element of beneficence. The intent of conducting research on innovative teaching strategies or examining how nursing students best learn is aimed at improving the quality of education, as well as students' outcomes. Although educators may view this as a beneficent act, students may not (Ridley, 2009). Individual students may not see the benefit of what they perceive to be a change from how they were previously taught. Additionally, there may be no educational gain for an individual student.

"Educational misconception" is another concern in that students may participate in a study because they believe that it will benefit them educationally (Leentjens & Levenson, 2013). They may believe that they will miss something educationally important if they are not part of the research. In addition, some students may be motivated by altruistic behaviors and agree to participate. Investigators need to be sensitive to these student perceptions and behaviors and incorporate strategies to minimize harm.

Protecting a participant's right to confidentiality is another important component of beneficence (Clark & McCann, 2005; Comer, 2009). The right to privacy is central to all research, and mechanisms need to be employed throughout the research process that minimize possible harm or risk for both those students who consent to participate and those who do not participate. Although most educational research is considered minimal risk, protection of the identity of participants must be well thought out (Heflin, DeMeo, Nagler, & Hockenberry, 2016). No matter the data collected, student identifiers or personal data, such as age, gender, race/ethnicity, must be protected. This is particularly true when data are collected on small numbers of students and their anonymity could be compromised.

The third moral requirement emphasized in the *Belmont Report* is *justice.* Justice is the idea of "fairness in distribution" (HHS, 1979, para. 19). Equitable selection and fair treatment of participants necessitates that the burdens of research should not be placed on any one particular group. Students are an accessible population for faculty and may not decline participation because of fear of adverse consequences (Comer, 2009). This potential ethical issue requires that investigators be clear in their research design that students are being invited to participate because they directly inform the research and answer the research questions.

Anderson (2011) argues for achieving a balance of the "valuable contribution of students as a resource with their potential vulnerability" (p. 30). Students are potentially in the best position to inform pedagogical practice since they are engaged participants in the teaching-learning process. Capturing their unique insights into knowledge development in a practice discipline and recognizing them as a new generation of learners, faculty need to be sensitive to maintaining the ethical integrity of the research and not exploiting the student's vulnerability in this context. Student perception of coercion and lack of autonomy is always a potential risk given the unequal power relationship (Anderson, 2011) and can create tensions in these dual roles for both the student and faculty (Shi, 2006). Strategies to minimize these perceptions and ensuring informed consent need to be based on the creation of a respectful and trusting environment.

Another aspect to this requirement of justice is that all eligible participants are given the opportunity to be in a study and none experience undue burden. The majority of research conducted in nursing education may have no direct benefit to the student, and this is something that needs to be clearly articulated in the consent process. In some instances, students may perceive themselves at a disadvantage in the classroom if they are not invited to participate in a research study (Bradbury-Jones & Alcock, 2010), particularly if the outcome is perceived as being desirable. This may create a challenge for investigators to balance the amount of information provided to participants to make an informed decision without confusing the participant and overburdening with extraneous information, giving the impression that there is a benefit.

Bradbury-Jones and Alcock (2010) provide a framework for ethical research practice to help investigators during the research process to make ethically sound decisions. The framework consists of three areas: research contribution, relationship, and impact (Bradbury-Jones & Alcock, 2010). The authors offer prompt questions in each area to provide investigators with direction during the research process. *Research contribution* questions focus on how a study will contribute to a body of knowledge that may benefit others in the future. It is incumbent on the investigator to be clear in the informed consent process that the student most likely will not experience the benefit of the research—in other words "no direct benefit"; however, the intent is to benefit nursing education. Suggesting to students that they may benefit from an innovative teaching strategy should not be stated and could be perceived as coercive. Providing sufficient information for the student to make an informed choice as to whether they want to participate is the best practice.

The second area of *research relationship* poses questions about the nature of the relationship between the student and investigator (Bradbury-Jones & Alcock, 2010). The focus is on being clear on the investigator's role as researcher and that the role is not one of a friend or counselor. Exploiting the research relationship is an example of a potential abuse of power. Mechanisms need to be in place to avoid undue pressure on the student participant.

Research impact is the third area of the framework (Bradbury-Jones & Alcock, 2010). Generally, most educational research is low in risk and does not involve physical harm; however, psychological effects, although minimal, may not be as apparent. For example, while interviewing nursing students who were unsuccessful in the clinical setting may provide important information to inform clinical education and provide some participants an opportunity to share their experience with an interested party, some may become emotionally distressed. Achieving a balance among research impact, research relationships, and potential risks is challenging. The questions presented in the ethical research practice framework can offer investigators guidance throughout the course of a research study.

Although common practice in some disciplines, it remains controversial whether students should be mandated to participate as research subjects in faculty research (Anderson, 2011; Leentjens & Levenson, 2013). Potential beneficial outcomes of research participation by students have been reported in the psychology and nursing literature. Rosell et al. (2005), in a study of 212 introductory psychology students, concluded that participation in the research process, as an active learning strategy, was an effective means of increasing research knowledge. In a longitudinal qualitative study of 13 undergraduate nursing students, Bradbury-Jones, Stewart, Irvine, and Sambrook (2011) reported three themes: strengthening self, strengthening knowledge, and strengthening clinical practice. Within the context of do no harm, they emphasized that in weighing the risks of educational research participation, investigators also need to be cognizant of possible benefits.

The *Belmont Report* (HHS, 1979) also addresses boundaries between practice and research, which are an important consideration in the educational setting. When an investigator departs from standard or usual pedagogical practice and implements a new innovative teaching strategy, the activity itself may not constitute research. Educators implement new strategies routinely to enhance and improve the learning experience for their students based on the context of the setting and the group of students. Thus, separating teaching practice from research can be challenging given the reciprocal relationship between the two processes. The point where the activity constitutes research is when the activity is "designed to test an hypothesis, permit conclusions to be drawn, and thereby to develop or contribute to generalizable knowledge" (HHS, 1979, para. 6). Since this distinction is not always clear, consultation with the investigator's IRB at this point may be warranted, as pedagogical practices and research often occur together.

Quality improvement (QI) projects designed to implement best teaching practices are another area where the distinction from a research activity is sometimes blurred (Keune et al., 2013). Regulatory oversight is mandatory for research to ensure the protection of human subjects; however, some institutions require local review of QI projects. With the proliferation of doctor of nursing practice projects, and some projects focusing on teaching practices, collaboration with one's IRB seems prudent. Protection of human subjects participating in QI projects and the translation of evidence is a relatively new area for many faculty guiding students conducting these projects and for the IRBs who may not be accustomed to reviewing them. Flow diagrams and report tools are available to assist in the decision-making process for investigators (Keune et al., 2013; Szanton, Taylor, & Terhaar, 2013). Allowing adequate time prior to the start of course or a QI project to make these determinations and obtain necessary approvals can alleviate any confusion and ensure protection of the human participants.

If any element in a project involves research, then review by an IRB is necessary (HHS, 1979). Investigators cannot assume their projects to be exempt because they are using a student population (Comer, 2009). DuBois (2002) argues, "as the name suggests, exempt research is still research" (p. 3), and the decision of whether a project is exempt rests with the IRB, not the investigator. Two basic elements of exempt research are that the participants' identities are protected and the risk is minimal. If there is any potential harm to the participant or there is any element of participant deception, the review may not be exempt. Even when a study is determined to be exempt, participant informed consent is required. Comprehensive decision trees for whether a study may be exempt or not are available online (www.hhs.gov/ohrp/policy/checklists/decisioncharts.html#).

Ethical Issues in Educational Research

Research conducted with human subjects is receiving greater scrutiny than ever (Sieber & Tolich, 2013). Scientific misconduct has been identified as an increasing concern in nursing publications and nursing science (Broome, Dougherty, Freda, Kearney, & Baggs, 2010; Fierz et al., 2014). Using the *Fostering Research Integrity in Europe* report, Fierz et al. (2014) reviewed available literature in nursing regarding research integrity promotion and concluded that scientific misconduct is a multilevel phenomenon and interventions must be targeted at every level. Data fabrication, data falsification, plagiarism, publication-related misconduct, failure to disclose conflicts of interest and ghostwriting, and authorship issues are examples of the types of misconduct that are occurring (Fierz et al., 2014). Although the authors acknowledge that the prevalence of some of these types of misconduct in nursing research is not specifically known, all investigators need to be cognizant of their existence.

Concerns of misconduct in research in nursing education are no different. The consequences of misconduct are far reaching, from the individual to the organizational and professional level. In the academic context, the pressure to conduct research and publish for promotion and tenure has the potential to impact scientific conduct. DuBois (2002) concluded that concerns of faculty self-promotion and the gain of individual benefits from educational research further support the requirement for human subjects review for research in this area. Research must have professional or societal value beyond the advancement of the investigator's career. To guard against any suggestion of impropriety, increasing the awareness and actions of investigators in the promotion of research integrity is crucial. Science is built on a foundation of societal trust (Committee on Science, Engineering, and Public Policy, 2009). The establishment of the scientific basis for the practice of nursing education depends on ethical behavior in all research practices.

Where in the research process can an investigator anticipate an ethical issue may occur? Ethical considerations have to be at the forefront of human subjects research, and the investigator needs to consider potential issues from conceptualization of a research study through dissemination of the findings (Creswell, 2014). This is true for all research designs, methods of data collection and analysis, contexts, and settings. To inform the practice of nursing education, investigators are collecting data most often from students since they best inform the teaching-learning process. Protecting their privacy starting with the research idea, prior to the study, through the reporting of the findings needs to take precedence in the investigator's mind.

Creswell (2014) identified five phases in the research process where potential ethical issues need to be anticipated: prior to conducting the study; beginning the study; collecting data; analyzing data; and reporting, sharing, and storing the data (Creswell, 2014, pp. 93–94). Each phase of the research process has its own ethical issues that should be considered, with possible ways to address them from an ethical framework. The process begins with exploring and examining basic ethical principles, professional association standards, and human subjects protection guidelines. In the final phase, one ethical behavior is to "report honestly" (Creswell, 2014, p. 94); a simple phrase that encompasses many of the elements of ethical scientific conduct.

As options in research design with respect to methods to recruit participants, data collection approaches (e.g., crowdsourcing, social media sites), analysis techniques (see Chapter 7), and dissemination choices (e.g., open access) change and expand, investigators are responsible for being informed and proactive in their research practices. To advance science, investigators sometimes have to take risks to explore innovative ideas, but "such risk taking does not excuse sloppy research . . . researchers have an obligation to the public, to their profession, and to themselves to be as accurate and careful as possible" (Committee on Science, Engineering, and Public Policy, 2009, p. 12).

The emerging area of data science warrants acknowledging another potential area of ethical issues for investigators conducting research in nursing education. The Council for Big Data, Ethics, and Society (http://bdes.datasociety.net), in collaboration with the National Science Foundation, is at the forefront of these discussions, helping to develop frameworks to assist investigators in understanding the implications of the big data phenomenon. The research landscape is changing, as multiple disciplines are employing big data research techniques to answer questions of relevance to their discipline. These techniques may use data that are in the public domain and available to anyone (sometimes for a fee), de-identified data, or data repositories (Metcalf, 2016). The challenges of big data and research ethics from a regulatory perspective are new to many fields, including nursing education. Conducting research using a big dataset requires investigators be knowledgeable about data science research and the relevant ethical issues. This is crucial as the science of nursing education advances.

Role of the Institutional Review Board

An IRB is the ethics gatekeeper (Shi, 2006) and provides a safety net for participants involved with research. This board advocates for the rights of humans involved in research. The IRB represents an independent group of five or more individuals who have been formally designated to approve, monitor, and review research involving humans with the aim to protect the rights and welfare of the study participants. The board is typically local to the setting and understands the research being conducted in that context. All IRBs must follow federal regulations; each may have unique considerations (Miser, 2005). To be considered legitimate, they must operate independently of the faculty governance structure (Oakes, 2002).

The OHRP (CFR, 2009) established basic requirements for review of applications and allows IRBs the latitude to use their judgment as to whether additional information would "meaningfully add to the protection of the rights and welfare of subjects" (§ 46.109). This is particularly relevant in regard to education research and the IRB's interpretation of regulations for consistency in application to protocols.

DuBois (2002) noted that for purposes of informed consent requirements in educational research, IRB consistency requires interpretation of what constitutes research versus assessment, a standard educational setting, and normal educational practice. Investigators may need guidance in these three areas as they relate to acquiring informed consent and protecting students' confidentiality or anonymity. Although research provides new generalizable knowledge, the research may subject the participants to some additional risk or burden beyond usual educational practice with no direct benefit. Additionally, research involves critical appraisal of its stated conclusions by peers through presentations, publications, and debate in the relevant body of literature.

From an ethical stance, compliance with IRB oversight should be seen as the "right thing to do" because it helps to protect the rights and welfare of the subjects of human research. In educational research, students are the human subjects. Balancing the protection of participants and their participation in research is difficult. Investigators are sometimes frustrated with the IRB review process, and some perceive IRBs as overstepping their role as protection of welfare and safety of participants and encroaching on faculty's academic freedom in the classroom (Thomson et al., 2013). Educating and working with one's IRB regarding research conducted in nursing education may help in alleviating some of the frustrations experienced and continue to provide the best protection for research participants. Most IRBs balance the concern about the rights of participants while being supportive of investigators and the need for advancing the science.

Engaging with the IRB to cultivate a positive relationship and ascertaining the best approaches within one's educational setting are prudent and worth the effort. Through qualitative interviews with 46 investigators, Cartwright, Hickman, Nelson, and Knafl (2013) identified key components for success in working with IRBs. Although the participants interviewed did not focus specifically on educational research, the findings are relevant to this discussion. The components to establishing a positive relationship included personal contact, proactive and ongoing communication, demonstrating expertise in one's area of research, minimizing the IRB's administrative burden and proactively seeking advice from the IRB, and careful attention to IRB policies and preferences regarding human subjects approval at their institutions (Cartwright et al., 2013). Application of the basic ethical principles to research in nursing education is discussed in the following section.

APPLICATION OF THE BASIC ETHICAL PRINCIPLES

Understanding and embracing the basic ethical principles that guide one's research practice is only the first step; application of these principles from start to finish in a research study is the challenge. Being proactive in the process can help to identify and minimize potential problems. Contact the IRB during the conceptualization and planning processes; this can strengthen the design of an effective educational study while yielding information that protects the research participants. Most universities have specific information regarding the IRB processes readily available on their home websites. Prior to starting a study, one should visit the IRB website and review the information provided. Talk with the IRB chair or representative to determine how educational research is handled at the institution. Table 6.1 includes specific suggestions to address and implement the ethical principles throughout a study in nursing education.

Three aspects of the research process are highlighted and further discussed here, as they often present a challenge to investigators. They are recruitment of participants, obtaining informed consent, and maintaining confidentiality and anonymity.

Recruitment of Participants

Students are learners in the academic setting, and as such, recruitment of them as research participants for a faculty member's research puts them in a vulnerable position, as discussed previously. Ideally, one should not use one's own students for research. Explore alternative strategies for recruiting a similar sample. Seeking participants from within the nursing program where the potential for direct interaction is minimal or from another institution certainly is preferable. Inherent in the nature of the educational setting, students may feel an obligation to participate, whether actual or perceived, because of a potential impact on grades and future letters of recommendation and relationships. Investigators should not use persuasion as a mechanism to encourage students to participate in their research. Unintentional or subliminal coercion needs to be avoided.

In the instance of employing one's own students for a research project, investigators should have an intermediary—someone not directly involved with the group—to conduct the recruitment. This individual needs to be cognizant of human subjects protection and not directly teaching the students so that any element or perception of coercion is avoided and the power differential is minimized. Possible options include colleagues teaching in other courses or research assistants. This individual could also be the contact person should the student participant decide to withdraw from a study. As noted by Ferguson et al. (2004), "reassuring students that they can withdraw at [any time] is moot if their decisions to participate in the first place are related to their dependency relationship with faculty" (p. 60). Additionally, maintaining the confidentiality of students who withdraw from the study is another important element.

Best practices for recruitment involve interested individuals contacting the investigator as opposed to the investigator directly approaching them. Providing potential participants with an information sheet that includes investigator contact information minimizes the possibility of coercion. This approach applies to recruitment flyers, email invitations, postings on social media sites, or other means of recruitment. These strategies can minimize the potential conflict of interest presented in the dual role of faculty and investigator.

TABLE 6.1

Ethical Issues in Research in Nursing Education

Phases of a Research Study	Recommendations to Address Potential Ethical Issues
Conceptualizing the study	<ul><li>Be proactive:<ul><li>Educate yourself about best practices in research ethics.</li><li>Consult with colleagues.</li><li>Get to know your IRB.</li><li>Thoroughly review the literature.</li><li>Search for funding opportunities.</li></ul></li><li>Begin networking:<ul><li>Explore partners within and outside one's own setting to assist with the research.</li><li>Select sites that best inform the research.</li></ul></li><li>Be certain that the population is most appropriate for the research purpose and questions.</li><li>Complete human subjects review certification.</li></ul>
Planning the study	<ul><li>Enlist a neutral individual external to the research to recruit, consent, collect data, and de-identify data.</li><li>Plan as if you are going to publish the research.</li><li>Partner with colleagues from other institutions.</li><li>Gain written permission to access the sites where data will be collected or participants recruited.</li><li>Consider potential psychological ramifications of research participation by the students and identify ways to minimize risk.</li><li>Put mechanisms in place to minimize potential investigator impact.</li><li>Create recruitment materials that are not coercive.</li><li>Complete the institutional review board (IRB) application in consultation with your IRB.</li></ul>
Recruiting participants	<ul><li>Recruit students outside of your own setting if at all possible.</li><li>Engage a neutral individual external to the research to recruit potential participants, particularly if they are your own students.</li><li>Do not offer extra credit, grade points, or preferential treatment during the recruitment process.</li></ul>
Obtaining written or implied consent	<ul><li>Identify oneself as an investigator for the research, not the teacher.</li><li>Disclose any potential conflicts of interest.</li><li>Engage a neutral individual external to the research to consent potential participants.</li><li>Be sure that your students understand what is standard education practice and what is research for the study.</li><li>Give students a copy of the consent form that clearly delineates how to withdraw should they choose to.</li><li>Clearly indicate during the consent process that not participating or leaving the study will not affect the course grade.</li><li>Allow sufficient time for the consent process.</li></ul>
Data collection and analysis	<ul><li>Collect data outside of class time.</li><li>Maintain the confidentiality of those students who do and do not participate.</li></ul>

TABLE 6.1	
Ethical Issues in Research in Nursing Education (*Continued*)	
Phases of a Research Study	**Recommendations to Address Potential Ethical Issues**
Dissemination of findings	• Maintain the confidentiality of participants through reporting of aggregate findings, recognizing potential identifiers, and use of pseudonyms. • Share findings with students and other colleagues through presentations and publications. • Report findings honestly.
Throughout the research process	• Role model ethical research behaviors. • Build trust through the use of ethical principles. • Serve on your IRB. • Mentor novice investigators. • Educate students and colleagues about the IRB and the research process.

Obtaining Informed Consent

Obtaining informed consent from participants is a crucial element of *respect for persons.* Understanding expectations of participation, independent choice, and opportunity to decide is central to informed consent. It should be clear in the consent that participation will not affect a student's grade or class standing. If investigators wish to use course assignments for research data, these data should not be accessed until final course grades have been submitted. It needs to be clearly stated in the consent and syllabus that the assignments are course requirements and represent standard educational practice; however, students have the option about participation in the research by allowing their assignments to be used for research.

Students may feel an obligation to participate in faculty research for the reasons articulated previously. Some may not fully and carefully read the consent form. Additionally, investing sufficient time in the consent process facilitates the development of a trusting relationship between student/participant and faculty/investigator. As with recruitment, every attempt to have an intermediary obtain consent should be employed.

Theiss, Hobbs, Giordano, and Brunson (2014) reported in a study of 60 undergraduate students that

> 80% of participants did not appear to read any portion of the consent form, or at least did not read carefully enough to recall the embedded instructions, [which] may reflect a flawed perception that consent forms are a mere formality in the research process. (p. 14).

As a best practice, they argue that investigators must minimize the impact of the "just sign here" culture and educate students in the meaning of giving informed consent. Investigators cannot assume understanding. Responsibility rests with investigators to allow adequate time to explain the consent to potential participants and build in a mechanism to ascertain understanding by participants. The notion that obtaining informed consent takes only 5 minutes of the participant's time is erroneous. As noted by Theiss et al. (2014), if students do not read the consent form, they are not truly giving informed consent.

In some instances, investigators may request a waiver of consent or the IRB may waive the requirement for a written consent form. These instances might include a retrospective review of student files or records that contain de-identified data or observations in a classroom. The research needs to involve no more than minimal risk of harm to the participant and could not practicably be carried out without a waiver. (Minimal risk means that the probability and magnitude of harm or discomfort anticipated in the research are not greater in and of themselves than those ordinarily encountered in daily life or during the performance of routine physical or psychological examinations or tests [CFR, 2009, § 46.102(i)]).

Waiver of a signature would also be considered if the written consent forms were the only record linking the participants and the research; the principal risk would be potential harm resulting from a breach of confidentiality (see CFR [2009] § 46.116 and § 46.117 for additional guidance on consent elements and waiver of consent).

A common example of a study where an investigator does not need signatures would be an anonymous online survey ascertaining students' perceptions or attitudes regarding their education. This waiver of a documented signed consent form, however, does not eliminate the need to inform participants of what they will be asked to do if they agree to participate in the study (Miser, 2005). Even in the case of implied consent, potential participants must be informed of all aspects of the nature of the research. The use of an informational sheet containing the basic elements of informed consent without the investigator obtaining a signature is necessary (see CFR [2009] § 46.116, General requirements for informed consent). The participant should receive a copy of this informational sheet.

Maintaining Confidentiality and Anonymity

Confidentiality and anonymity are based on the ethical principle of *respect*. Protecting the student's right to confidentiality needs to be considered in all aspects of the research process. It is the student's decision as to what is shared; the student controls the context and extent of that information. There is a direct relationship between the need for privacy and the sensitivity of the information being collected. Issues concerning privacy can occur during recruitment in how potential participants are identified, as well as during data collection and reporting. For example, in a study exploring how students feel after a clinical failure, investigators directly approaching students who have failed to participate violates their right to privacy. Depending on the sensitivity of the research topic, such as clinical failure, a focus group may not be the best way collect data and protect a student's privacy. Likewise, this principle of respect includes protecting a student's privacy should they decide to withdraw from a study.

Confidentiality extends privacy to the management and access of identifiable data by investigators to the information that the student has shared in the research process. Access to data should be limited to only designated individuals involved in the study. Any breach of confidentiality can compromise trust in the research process and influence the teaching-learning process. Maintaining confidentiality in qualitative research studies adds further challenges when direct quotes or personal stories are used as exemplars of the findings. Investigators need to ensure that the reporting of the findings is sensitive to the extent that the release of data could harm a student, and strategies to protect privacy must be considered. Special attention must be paid to the reporting of demographic data in qualitative research given the fewer participants. Collecting data on gender may have similar implications, and to protect a male student's privacy, his identity and responses should be pooled with the other responses.

The most effective means to ensure privacy for the student participant is collecting data anonymously, whether by paper and pencil or electronically. If the investigator cannot link the research data to any specific participant, anonymity can be guaranteed. When data are collected at multiple time periods, such as with a pretest and posttest, this means creating a mechanism to code data for the purpose of linking questionnaires. Explaining this process of coding to students is important so that they understand that their data, once collected, cannot be removed from the study. When collecting data electronically, the investigator needs to be well informed of the mechanisms in place with the online survey services that maintain the privacy and security of the data. The validity of data will more likely be enhanced if the investigator implements strategies to maintain students' privacy.

CONCLUSIONS AND IMPLICATIONS

To generate empirical evidence for nursing education practice, research with those who best inform the teaching-learning process will be the students. The strength of involving students is that they can provide fresh insight and have the student voice (Anderson, 2011). However, investigators must acknowledge that students are valuable and vulnerable (Anderson, 2011). Students need to be well informed to protect their rights as research participants. Being a role model as an investigator and demonstrating good research habits could provide an opportunity to educate students in research ethics and reinforces trust in the research process (DuBois, 2002). In this age of evidence-based teaching practice, debriefing sessions about the IRB and research process can only strengthen the science and teaching-learning outcomes. Trust and the basic ethical principles of *respect, beneficence,* and *justice* are the foundation of both the research and educational process.

The research community as a whole suffers when even a few investigators ignore basic principles of ethics and proceed without adequate safeguards. Society entrusts investigators with the privilege of using human subjects to advance scientific knowledge and expects investigators to show respect for research subjects. However, investigators bear the ultimate ethical responsibility for their work with human subjects; best practice in protecting research participants is the right thing to do.

ACKNOWLEDGMENTS

I thank my colleagues on the IRB at Widener University for the ongoing dialogue about best practices in conducting research in a higher education context. In particular, I wish to acknowledge Bob Wellmon and Angie McNelis for the many engaging conversations we had that focused on the protection of the rights of human subjects. Their insights were invaluable.

References

American Educational Research Association. (2015). *What is education research?* Retrieved June 10, 2016, from http://www.aera.net/EducationResearch/WhatisEducationResearch/tabid/13453/Default.aspx

American Nurses Association. (2015). *Code of ethics for nurses with interpretive statements.* Silver Spring, MD: Nursesbooks.org.

Anderson, G. (2011). Students as valuable but vulnerable participants in research: Getting the balance right using a feminist approach and focus group interviews. *Evidence Based Midwifery, 9*(1), 30–34.

Aycock, D., & Currie, E. (2013). Minimizing risks for nursing students recruited for health and educational research. *Nurse Educator, 38,* 56–60. doi:10.1097/NNE.0b013e3182829c3a

Bradbury-Jones, C., & Alcock, J. (2010). Nursing students as research participants: A framework for ethical practice. *Nurse Education Today, 30,* 192–196. doi:10.1016/j.nedt.2009.07.013

Bradbury-Jones, C., Stewart, S., Irvine, F., & Sambrook, S. (2011). Nursing students' experiences of being a research participant: Findings from a longitudinal study. *Nurse Education Today, 31,* 107–111. doi:10.1016/j.nedt.2010.04.006

Broome, M. E., Dougherty, M. C., Freda, M. C., Kearney, M. H., & Baggs, J. G. (2010). Ethical concerns of nursing reviewers: An international survey. *Nursing Ethics, 17,* 741–748. doi:10.1177/0969733010379177

Cartwright, J., Hickman, S., Nelson, C., & Knafl, K. (2013). Investigators' successful strategies for working with institutional review boards. *Research in Nursing and Health, 36,* 478–486. doi:10.1002/nur.21553

Clark, E., & McCann, T. (2005). Researching students: An ethical dilemma. *Nurse Researcher, 12*(3), 42–50. doi:10.7748/nr2005.01.12.3.42.c5947

Cleary, M., Walter, G., & Jackson, D. (2014). Above all, 'do no harm': Key considerations when including students as research participants in higher education settings. *Contemporary Nurse, 49,* 93–95. doi:10.1080/10376178.2014.11081958

Code of Federal Regulations. (2009). Protection of human subjects, 45 C.F.R. Retrieved June 10, 2016, from http://www.hhs.gov/ohrp/policy/ohrpregulations.pdf

Comer, S. (2009). The ethics of conducting educational research on your own students. *Journal of Nursing Law, 13,* 100–105. doi:10.1891/1073-7472.13.4.100

Committee on Science, Engineering, and Public Policy. (2009). *On being a scientist: A guide to responsible conduct in research* (3rd ed.). Washington, DC: National Academies Press.

Creswell, J. W. (2014). *Research design: Qualitative, quantitative, and mixed methods approaches* (4th ed.). Thousand Oaks, CA: Sage.

DuBois, J. (2002). When is informed consent appropriate in educational research? Regulatory and ethical issues. *IRB: Ethics and Human Research, 24*(1), 1–8.

Ferguson, L., Yonge, O., & Myrick, F. (2004). Students' involvement in faculty research: Ethical and methodological issues. *International Journal of Qualitative Methods, 3*(4), Article 5. Retrieved June 10, 2016, from http://www.ualberta.ca/~iiqm/backissues/3_4/pdf/ferguson.pdf

Fierz, K., Gennaro, S., Dierickx, K., Van Achterberg, T., Morin, K. H., De Geest, S., et al. (2014). Scientific misconduct: Also an issue in nursing science?. *Journal of Nursing Scholarship, 46,* 271–280. doi:10.1111/jnu.12082

Gresley, R. S. (2009). Building a science of nursing education. In C. Schultz (Ed.), *Building a science of nursing education: Foundation for evidence-based teaching-learning* (pp. 1–13). New York: National League for Nursing.

Heflin, M., DeMeo, S., Nagler, A., & Hockenberry, M. (2016). Health professions education research and the institutional review board. *Nurse Educator, 41*(2), 55–59. doi:10.1097/NNE.0000000000000230

Keune, J., Brunsvold, M., Hohmann, E., Korndorffer, J., Weinstein, D., & Smink, D. (2013). The ethics of conducting graduate medical education research on residents. *Academic Medicine, 88*, 449–453. doi:10.1097/ACM.0b013e3182854bef

Kirkwood, K. (2012). The professor really wants me to do my homework: Conflicts of interest in educational research. *American Journal of Bioethics, 12*(4), 47–48. doi:10.1080/15265161.2012.656813

Leentjens, A., & Levenson, J. (2013). Ethical issues concerning recruitment of university students as research subjects. *Journal of Psychosomatic Research, 75*, 394–398. doi:10.1016/j.jpsychores.2013.03.007

Metcalf, J. (2016). Human-subjects protections and big data: Open questions and changing landscapes. *Council for Big Data, Ethics, and Society.* Retrieved June 10, 2016, from http://bdes.datasociety.net/council-output/human-subjects-protections-and-big-data-open-questions-and-changing-landscapes/

Miser, W. (2005). Educational research: To IRB, or not to IRB?. *Family Medicine, 37*, 168–173.

Oakes, J. M. (2002). Risks and wrongs in social science research: An evaluator's guide to the IRB. *Evaluation Review, 26*, 443–479. doi:10.1177/019384102236520

Resnik, D. B. (2011). What is ethics in research and why is it important? *National Institute of Environmental Health Sciences.* Retrieved June 10, 2016, from http://www.niehs.nih.gov/research/resources/bioethics/whatis/

Ridley, R. (2009). Assuring ethical treatment of students as research participants. *Journal of Nursing Education, 48*, 537–541. doi:10.3928/01484834-20090610-08

Rosell, M. C., Beck, D. M., Luther, K. E., Goedert, K. M., Shore, W. J., & Anderson, D. D. (2005). The pedagogical value of experimental participation paired with course content. *Teaching of Psychology, 32*(2), 95–99. doi:10.1207/s15328023top3202_3

Shi, L. (2006). Students as research participants or learners?. *Journal of Academic Ethics, 4*, 205–220. doi:10.1007/s10805-006-9028-y

Sieber, J., & Tolich, M. B. (2013). *Planning ethically responsible research* (2nd ed.). Thousand Oaks, CA: Sage.

Szanton, S., Taylor, H., & Terhaar, M. (2013). Development of an institutional review board preapproval process for doctor of nursing practice students: Process and outcome. *Journal of Nursing Education, 52*, 51–55. doi:10.3928/01484834-20121212-01

Theiss, J., Hobbs, W., Giordano, P., & Brunson, O. (2014). Undergraduate consent form reading in relation to conscientiousness, procrastination, and point-of-time effect. *Journal of Empirical Research on Human Research Ethics, 9*(3), 11–17. doi:10.1177/1556264614540593

Thomson, J., Elgin, C., Hyman, D., Schrag, Z., Knight, J., & Kreiser, B. R. (2013). *Regulation of research on human subjects: Academic freedom and the institutional review board* (Subcommittee Final Report). Washington, DC: American Association of University Professors.

U.S. Department of Health and Human Services. (1979). *The Belmont Report: Ethical principles and guidelines for the protection of human subjects of research.* Retrieved June 10, 2016, from http://www.hhs.gov/ohrp/humansubjects/guidance/belmont.html

7

Managing, Analyzing, and Interpreting Data

Karen H. Morin, PhD, RN, FAAN, ANEF

Investigators are always happy when data have been collected and they can turn their energy toward analyzing and interpreting what the data offer relative to study research questions or hypotheses. For most investigators, this phase of research is the most enjoyable, as the end of this particular research effort is in sight. Nonetheless, this phase in not without potential pitfalls and issues. The purposes of this chapter are to highlight best practices in data management, analysis, and interpretation, and to discuss future trends in data analysis.

Such a discussion is essential, given current concerns about the quality of research about nursing education. Experts in nursing education increasingly are more vocal about the need to produce high-quality research (Ironside & Spurlock, 2014; Morin, 2013, 2014; St. Pierre Schneider, Nicholas, & Kumas, 2013; Valiga & Ironside, 2012). Not only are there concerns about the quality of research exploring nursing education issues, there also is considerable cross-disciplinary discussion about the need for the responsible conduct of research (RCR) (Kalichman, Sweet, & Plemmons, 2014, 2015; Ulrich, Wallen, Cui, Chittmans, Sweet, & Plemmons, 2015). Investigators interested in nursing education issues who are familiar with actions associated with scientific misconduct, such as data fabrication, data falsification, and plagiarism (FFP), that have propelled these discussions (Fierz et al., 2014; John, Loewenstein, & Prelec, 2012; Fanelli, 2009; Sijtsma, 2015). However, they may be less familiar with questionable research practices (QRPs), those practices that fall between RCR and FFP. Several of these QRPs fall within the realm of the topic of this chapter. For example, Sijtsma (2015, para 3) highlighted practices such as "ignoring the influence of outliers on statistical results" and "stepwise increasing the sample" as being of questionable practice. A more comprehensive list is presented in Box 7.1. These practices can range on a continuum from purely innocent to clearly fraudulent (Sijtsma, 2015).

Moreover, because public and investigator concerns have been prevalent, the U.S. Department of Health and Human Services Office of Research Integrity published a "comprehensive overview of basic rules of the road for responsible research" (Steneck, 2007, p. v). Although the audience for this resource is beginning investigators, as well as small to mid-size research institutions, investigators investigating nursing education questions may find Chapters 6 and 8 particularly helpful when undertaking data management, analysis, and reporting.

BOX 7.1

Data Reporting Problems in the Scientific Literature

Failing to include the number of eligible participants
Inaccurately reporting missing data points
Failing to report all pertinent data
Failing to report negative results
Allowing research sponsors to influence reporting of results
Inappropriately labeling graphs
Reporting percentages rather than actual numbers
Using and reporting inappropriate statistical tests
Reporting differences when statistical significance is not reached
Reporting no difference when power is inadequate
Failing to correct for multiple comparisons; data dredging
Splitting data into multiple publications
Inappropriately using terms lacking precise language
Reporting findings not supported by the data
Ignoring citations or prior work that challenge study conclusions
Inflating research results for the media

(Adapted with permission from Marco, C. A., & Larkin, G. L. (2006). Research ethics: Ethical issues of data reporting and the quest for authenticity. *Academic Emergency Medicine, 7*, 691–694.)

Implementing data management, analysis, and interpretation strategies based on best practice and a clear understanding of what constitutes RCR and QRP can contribute to ensuring that information is presented accurately. Following best practices, then, can contribute to moving forward the development of the science of nursing education. Importantly, best practices are applicable, *irrespective of the type of research conducted* (qualitative, quantitative, or multimethod). Moreover, no discussion of data management, analysis, and interpretation is adequate without acknowledging the critical role played by posing relevant research questions, using appropriate designs and instruments (when applicable), and acknowledging theoretical underpinnings of the study. Data management, collection, and analysis cannot address findings when fatal flaws are present in a study. Irrelevant research questions yield irrelevant analyses and interpretation.

What then are the best practices when dealing with data? For clarity, information is presented by stage of the research process. Best practices in data management, data analysis, and interpretation are typically discussed in the Methodology section of a research proposal or report.

DATA MANAGEMENT

Data management strategies and issues should be determined prior to the collection of data (Macrina, 2014; Steneck, 2007). Thus, investigators need to be clear about ownership of the data, how data are collected and stored, and with whom and how data will be shared (Steneck, 2007). Unfortunately, this step, "crucial to scientific research" (Macrina, 2014, p. 329),

TABLE 7.1

Best Practices for Individual Investigators

Useful data books explain:	*Good data books:*
• What you did	• Are legible and written in ballpoint pen ink
• Why you did it	• Are well organized and up-to-date
• How you did it	• Are accurate and complete
• When you did it	• Include data output affixed to pages (e.g., photos, transcripts)
• Where materials are	• Allow repetition of your work
• What happened (and what did not happen)	• Are compliant with relevant funding agency and institutional requirements
• Your interpretations	• Are accessible to authorized person, stored properly, and appropriately backed up
• Contributions of others	• Are properly witnessed when necessary
• What's next	• Are properly recognized as the property of your institution
	• Are the ultimate record of your scientific contributions

SOURCE: Reprinted with permission from Macrina, F. L. (2014). Scientific record keeping. In F. L. Macrina (Ed.). *Scientific integrity. Text and cases in responsible conduct of research* (4th ed., p. 330). Washington, DC: American Society for Microbiology. © 2014 American Society for Microbiology. Used with permission. No further reproduction or distribution is permitted without prior written permission of American Society for Microbiology.

is often overlooked in research training, as well as by investigators. Nonetheless, "good record keeping fosters the scientific norms of accuracy, replication, and reliability" (Macrina, 2014, p. 331). There are excellent research reasons for this, and additionally, good record keeping has legal implications. Funders may audit records, and questionable record keeping could lead to funding being discontinued or declined. Good record keeping is critical when addressing questions of research misconduct. Investigators want to ensure that their data records are complete, secure, link types of data to each other (e.g., linking paper code book to electronic records), are reviewed on a regular basis (weekly or monthly), and accurately reflect all research activities (Macrina, 2014).

Although investigators may desire a prescriptive approach to data management, Macrina (2014) argues that there are a variety of correct approaches. What investigators need to keep in mind are the key foundational best practices to guide individual investigator data management, which are presented in Table 7.1. Scheier, Wilson, and Resnik (2006) expanded these practices beyond those for individual investigators to include best practices for research team leaders (Box 7.2), departments or schools, and academic institutions. Granted that these best practices are offered from a basic science perspective, much of the discussion related to these best practices is relevant to nursing education scientists. Specific best practices are discussed in the following paragraphs.

Define the Data

Readers may consider the best practice of defining data to be self-evident. Do not all investigators explicate what constitutes data in a study? Why the need to emphasize this best practice? Macrina (2014) states that data "are any form of factual information used for reasoning" (p. 332). Thus, there are many forms of data (Macrina, 2014). Moreover, data can be tangible (e.g., biological samples, questionnaires, examination

---

BOX 7.2

Best Practices for Leaders of Research Groups

Research group leaders should:

- Set standards for record keeping regarding:
  - Research study/activities, e.g., handwritten or electronic notes
  - Labeling samples, tangible products
- How communication is conveyed [minutes of meetings, etc.]
- Provide/assure team training in record keeping
- Articulate benefits and consequences of record keeping
- Share examples of good record keeping
- Periodically review team member records
- Stipulate ownership of data and records
- Make available tools for record keeping [hard copy or electronic]
- Hold team members accountable for maintaining standards
- Encourage sharing of project information amongst team members
- Have a transition plan for when members leave the team
- Assure compliance with other institutional and legal requirements
- Develop a process by which data can be accessed for a pre-determined time period

---

Source: Reprinted with permission from Scheier, A. A., Wilson, K., & Resnik, D. (2006). Academic research record-keeping: Best practices for individuals, group leaders, and institutions. *Academic Medicine, 81,* 42–47.

---

scores, transcripts) and intangible (field notes, written notes in a data book). Identifying appropriate data is essential, as the type of data collected affects data analysis. Identifying this information is critical when considering replication of studies (more on replication will be presented later in this chapter).

The following example reinforces the many types of data possible in a study. A doctoral student wished to determine whether a cultural sensitivity intervention enhances senior students' cultural sensitivity. In addition to administering an established cultural assessment instrument, the doctoral student gathered data about participant reflections following a matching card game, viewing a video, and at the end of the day-long intervention. Participants also were asked to "free write" following a lecture. Finally, the doctoral student conducted individual participant interviews following participant graduation. Identification of the many types of data gathered in this study required considerable discussion with committee members over a prolonged period of time.

Establish Who Owns the Data

Data ownership is critical to scientific integrity. Nursing education scientists may question the emphasis on this best practice, as ownership issues are frequently discussed in relation to funding agencies or organizations (Steneck, 2007). Given the dearth of funding opportunities for research addressing nursing education questions, ownership of the data may be considered a moot point. Yet discussion of ownership is equally relevant when undertaking collaborative research with other nurse scientists or scientists from other disciplines. For example, an evaluator who is skilled in data analysis and external to the organization may be hired, and this person manipulates all of the data (data entry, cleaning, analysis). Consequently, this person has a complete set of data, along with the original data (e.g., questionnaires). What does this person do with the data? Certainly, raw data may be returned to the principal investigator (PI), but what happens to the data file? Is it returned to the PI, or does the evaluator retain it? The PI needs to make explicit that ownership of all data (original and computer generated) rests with the PI; thus, a reasonable expectation is that all data are returned to the PI.

"Research subjects and entities that have or can be the source of important data may no longer be willing to provide or be the source of data without some ownership stake in the end results" (Steneck, 2007, p. 90). Thus, ownership of data is often shared with communities of interest, such as when conducting community-based participatory research (CBPR) (Minkler, 2005). Last, an important practice is to seek clarification relative to institutional ownership of data. Investigations of student service-learning outcomes, specifically those developed in collaboration with a community, is an example of CBPR.

Establish Sound Record-Keeping Practices

As with other best practices, sound record keeping provides for transparency in all aspects of the research project and serves as evidence in the event that findings are questioned. Thus, data recording processes are established prior to data collection. The following traditional data recording methods have been challenged with the advent of technologies such as computerized programs (e.g., Microsoft® Excel), the increasing presence of research teams, and the use of self-reporting instruments (Scheier et al., 2006). Although these advancements may benefit science, they contribute to "the physical fragmentation of research records" (Scheier et al., 2006, p. 43) and limit data record oversight. Investigators should keep these limitations in mind as they stipulate record-keeping practices.

Data should be recorded in some sort of data book; the form can be either paper or electronic (Macrina, 2014; Steneck, 2007). The following suggestions are offered within the perspective of basic science practices. Nonetheless, they reflect excellent practices and are transferable to research conducted in nursing education.

When using a paper data book, consider the following: (a) use acid-free paper to guarantee permanence; (b) limit exposure to strong sunlight, humidity, excessive temperatures, and dust; (c) use a ballpoint black ink pen to record information; and (d) use either a bound or loose-leaf binder in which to store all data. Electronic record-keeping practices warrant special discussion, given the potential for data records to be compromised by individuals not associated with the study (Macrina, 2014). A summary of appropriate best practices related to electronic records is presented in Box 7.3.

One of the primary roles of the investigator is to determine with whom data books will be shared. Investigators addressing nursing education issues often undertake research alone. However, the push for collaborative disciplinary and interdisciplinary research means that nursing education scientists will be interacting with other scientists and team members. Thus, maintaining a record of who has access to the data is critical. For example, an investigator agrees to work with a doctoral student for a semester to help meet the student's research requirements. As part of the work, the student will have

---

BOX 7.3

Sound Electronic Record-Keeping Practices

- Identify the custodian of the records
- Define what constitutes electronic records
- Explicate organization and storage location
- Encrypt and write protect stored data
- Time stamp data to ensure authenticity
- Back up data on a regular basis
- Limit access to the data (principal investigator and who else?)

(Adapted with permission from Macrina, F. L. (2014). Scientific record keeping. In F. L. Macrina (Ed.). *Scientific integrity. Text and cases in responsible conduct of research* (4th ed., pp. 346–347). Washington, DC: ASM Press.)

---

access to the data book—recall the data book contains all study data. The investigator should note separately the date, student name, and project associated with access to the data book.

Clarify How Data Will Be Stored

Explicating how data will be stored prior to data collection is another important best practice. An essential aspect of this practice is familiarity with the requirements of the funding agency or academic institution. For example, data must be retained for at least 3 years if funded by the National Institutes of Health. However, individual academic or health care entities may stipulate a longer time period. Current thinking among scientists is that data should never be destroyed, as having access to data could enhance replication (Hubbard, 2016).

Summary

Best practices for data management exist (Macrina, 2014; Scheier et al., 2006; Stenick, 2007; Strasser, Cook, Michener, & Buddin, n.d.) and are summarized visually in Figure 7.1. Armed with these best practices, nursing education scientists can initiate the appropriate processes and policies to ensure that guidelines are employed as they undertake analysis of data gathered to address relevant and pressing nursing education research questions.

DATA ANALYSIS AND INTERPRETATION

Undertaking the analysis of data, with concomitant interpretation, can be most rewarding. However, a cursory review of QRP, presented in Table 7.1, reveals that data analysis and interpretation is often an area where QRP may arise. Moreover, these practices are not limited to one specific research approach. However, for ease of presentation, best practices by type of research approach will be discussed.

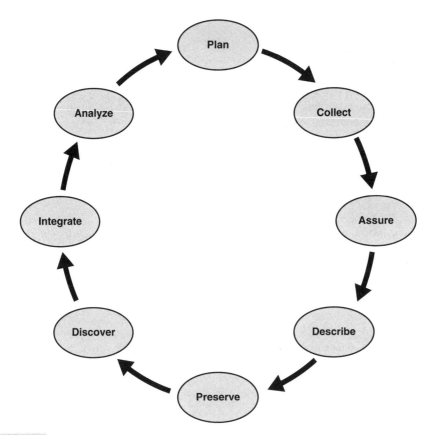

FIGURE 7.1 *The data life cycle.* Reprinted with permission from: Strasser, C., Cook, R., Michener, W., & Buddin, A. (2012). Primer on data management: What you always wanted to know. A DataONE publication. http://dx.doi.org/doi:10.5060/D2251G48

Best Practices for Quantitative Analysis

Best practices for quantitative analysis include using a statistician, respecting missing data, avoiding hypothesizing once the results are known, and ensuring that theory is used to guide analysis.

Use a Statistician

Certainly, nurse scientists have training in statistics; however, statistics is not generally their area of expertise. Just as a nurse scientist would think nothing of inviting colleagues from education or sociology to join their research team, so also should they include statisticians as part of the research team. In fact, best practice is to include them when initial discussion of the research project begins and issues are identified. Statisticians can provide input on study design, help clarify the research questions, and preemptively highlight potential issues with data analysis (Hayat, Higgins, Schwartz, & Staggs, 2015;

Hayat, Schmiege, & Cook, 2014). Their role in identifying the correct statistical tests is essential to ensuring findings are interpreted appropriately.

Many investigators undertaking research about nursing education work in nonresearch environments and may argue that access to a statistician is limited, if not impossible. Nonetheless, best practice provides the impetus to reach out to colleagues with statistical expertise in other departments within their institution or outside their institution. Doing so enhances the knowledge contributions made by their research efforts.

Treat Missing Data With Respect

Best practice in data analysis calls for the accurate reporting of missing data, yet Horner and Minifie (2011) and Marco and Larken (2000) have documented how missing data have been reported has been suspect. Investigators are reminded that "missing data must be accounted for in data analysis in order for researchers to draw valid conclusions" (Jeličić, Phelps, & Lerner, 2009, p. 1196). Not accounting for missing data also contributes to violations of statistical tests employed in a study. Earlier practices for treating missing data, such as deleting cases or single-value mean substitution, are no longer appropriate, as they result in the underestimation of variances and standard errors, contributing to biased results (Jeličić et al., 2009). Newer methods based on statistical theory and a theoretical framework for missing data estimates are available. They include multiple imputation, direct maximum likelihood, and full information maximum likelihood (Jeličić et al., 2009). Investigators can enhance the presentation of their analysis by reporting missing values for each variable studied, sharing thoughts on possible reasons for missing data, or articulating how missing data were treated. Doing so fosters transparency of the research process.

Avoid Hypothesizing After the Results Are Known

According to Kerr (1998), *hypothesizing after the results are known* (HARKing) is the presentation of "a post hoc hypothesis in the introduction of a research report as if it were an a priori hypothesis" (p. 197). In other words, an investigator, having determined that the original hypothesis was not significant, performs a series of additional analysis in the hope of obtaining significant results. Should the investigator be successful, which is highly likely given the galloping alpha effect, then only those findings are presented (Spellman, 2013). Kline (2013), in fact, urges investigators to avoid inventing a rationale for performing a fishing expedition in search of significant findings. Similarly, investigators may be tempted to continue sampling until analysis of findings reveals significance. HARKing and continued sampling are practices to be avoided, as they threaten scientific integrity of investigator research efforts.

Interestingly, a related concern has surfaced in relation to qualitative analysis. Recently, an established investigator indicated, during a conversation with a doctoral student, that the resulting analysis of qualitative data may require changing the initial research question. Further discussion with experts in qualitative research would indicate that such a practice is not totally uncommon. In essence, this practice—changing the question to match the findings—is the qualitative version of HARKing. Such a practice should be avoided.

Use Theory to Guide Analysis

When possible, theory should drive how data are analyzed. Yet frequently, such is not the case. A cursory review of nursing education publications reinforces the need to employ this best practice more consistently. Such best practice is applicable irrespective of type of research conducted. As Sandelowski (2010) so eloquently states, "No study of any kind could ever be so conceptually naked" (p. 79), even when a theory is not explicitly discussed.

Best Practices for Qualitative Analysis

Best practices for qualitative analysis include focusing on how data answer the research question driving the study and explicating how rigor is maintained in analyzing the data.

Be True to the Research Question

The best practice of being true to the research question relates to how qualitative investigators analyze data. The focus should be on how the data answer the research question that was the driver for the study. As data are analyzed, using well-established methods explicated by such authorities as Miles, Huberman, and Saldaña (2014) and Marshall and Rossman (2016), the investigator keeps the overarching research questions in mind. Although there may be times when data do not answer the overarching questions, to not acknowledge such as situation would be a misrepresentation of the original purpose of the study.

Explicating How Rigor Is Maintained

Qualitative data analysis takes considerably more time than quantitative analysis. Best practice involves allowing sufficient time to "live with the data." Tong, Sainsbury, and Craig (2007) reinforce the need to be specific about the number of coders, how data are coded, and how themes are derived and identified. How trustworthiness of the data has been established should be transparent.

FUTURE ANALYTIC METHODS

Scientists in many disciplines, such as medicine, psychology, social science, and business, are calling for reconceptualizing how quantitative, but not qualitative, research findings can be made more useful and relevant (Hubbard, 2016). This reconceptualization will require a paradigmatic shift in how investigators approach knowledge generation, what they consider constitutes science, and what constitutes empirical generalizations. Hubbard argues that empirical generalizations—that is, "results . . . repeatable over a wide range of conditions (e.g., organizations, geographic areas, time periods, measurement instruments, methods of data collection, researchers)" (p. 3)—are sorely lacking in his disciplinary literature, social and management sciences. Such an observation is equally applicable to research in nursing education in that there are few empirical generalizations. Moreover, Hubbard argues it is only when empirical generalizations are present that knowledge is advanced.

Hubbard (2016) attributes the absence of empirical generalizations to an overwhelming endorsement of "one single methodological paradigm, one that revolves around the idea of significant difference" (p. 4). This paradigm diminishes a discipline's ability to generate facts and to develop theories driven by these facts. Rather, it fosters the quick development and testing of theories using the hypothetico-deductive model of explanation. Thus, the goal of research efforts within this paradigm is to achieve statistically significant ($p < .05$) results. Although investigators embracing this paradigm (of which there are many!) strive for research that is innovative, doing so typically does not add to what is known about a particular phenomenon. Moreover, investigators use unique datasets, do not consider external validity issues such as generalization, and tend to "overgeneralize their results to other contexts or time periods" (Hubbard, 2016, p. 5). The outcome of such a paradigm is that investigators have a series of unique study findings indicating differences, but how these study findings are similar is unclear. The lack of clarity limits the advancement of knowledge. Moreover, the significant difference paradigm views "knowledge procurement as instantaneous, brought about by the unquestioning application of formal statistical protocols looking for $p < .05$ results in single-shot studies" (Hubbard, 2016, p. 69).

Cumming (2012), Kline (2013), and Hubbard (2016) advocate another paradigm, one that emphasizes significant sameness. In this paradigm, emphasis is on unearthing observed regularities that lead to generalizations that are deeper and higher (Hubbard, 2016). This paradigm reinforces that thinking about knowledge is neither easy nor prescribed but rather is messy. Hubbard (2016) asserts:

> Data rarely speak for themselves; universal generalizations are impossible because of the intrinsically contingent nature of relationships; and model uncertainty is a fact of life and cannot be addressed by even the most sophisticated statistical manipulations in a single data set, but which can be resolved by gathering additional data via well-designed studies. (p. 5)

This paradigm asserts that uncertainty is inherent in knowledge generation and that knowledge generation is undertaken over time in research programs. Such a perspective challenges how the majority of nurse scientists have been educated relative to the conduct of research and interpretation of data using statistical tests.

The significant sameness paradigm also challenges investigators' continuing reliance on null hypothesis significance testing (NHST) as the only way to assess hypotheses and arrive at conclusions. This reliance fosters dichotomous thinking, presenting investigators with having to make an "either-or" decision (Cumming, 2012), implies that the result is absolute rather than provisional (Hubbard, 2016), and impedes knowledge development (Kline, 2013). Unfortunately, the test of significance, reflective of the significant difference paradigm, has become the critical underpinning of all that is research, from design to dissemination (Hubbard, 2016). Moreover, in this paradigm, "statistical inference and scientific inference are interchangeable; asterisks outweigh substance" (Hubbard, 2016, p. 31). The significant sameness model is one effort to counter the pervasiveness of the NHST. A comparison of paradigm characteristics is presented in Box 7.4.

Criticisms of NHST are not new. Increasingly, cognitive errors engendered by this approach are questioned, as scientists in all disciplines recognize the need for reproducible research (Asendorpf et al., 2013; Laine, Goodman, Griswold, & Sox, 2007). Research

BOX 7.4

Comparison of Significant Sameness and Significant Difference Paradigms

Significant Sameness

- **Conception of knowledge:** Problematic, messy, and requires weeding out errors
- **Model of Science:** Theory developed using induction based on empirical regularities using many datasets; abductive inference key; requires many studies over time; generalizations are restricted, not generalizations supported by extensive empirical findings "and known boundary conditions" (p. 8)
- **Negative results:** Essential to boundary setting, and better theory
- **Importance of replication:** Crucial to paradigm; supports validity generalization process
- **Replication defined:** Overlapping confidence intervals
- **View of generalization:** "Empirical generalizations across data sets" (p. 8)
- **Model uncertainty:** Uncertainty readily acknowledged, with statistics taking a subordinate role to research design
- **Nature of predictions:** Predictive prediction and severe tests critical; quantitative
- **Role of p-values:** Not an objective measure of knowledge, less emphasis
- **Role of effect sizes:** Regularly reported and interpreted
- **Role of confidence intervals:** Regularly reported and interpreted
- **Investigator Philosophy:** Focused on knowledge development

Significant Difference

- **Conception of knowledge** is unproblematic, focus on rejecting [null] hypothesis at p < .05
- **Model of Science:** Focused on testing rather than developing theory, reflective of logical positivist approach to science; one study produces "rational knowledge" (p. 7); universal generalizations produced by good theory
- **Negative results:** Rarely shared (published)
- **Importance of replication:** Considered as inferior research; emphasis in on novel research
- **Replication defined:** "Statistical significance in same direction as earlier study" (8)
- **View of generalization:** From sample to population, with reliance on random sampling
- **Model uncertainty:** Typically ignored, reinforcing primacy of statistics in knowledge generation
- **Nature of predictions:** Qualitative
- **Role of p-values:** Considered critical to establish knowledge claims
- **Role of effect sizes:** Not consistently reported and interpreted
- **Role of confidence intervals:** Rarely reported in business or nursing education disciplines
- **Investigator Philosophy:** Knowledge development secondary to personal career advancement

Source: Reprinted from *Journal of Business Research, 66(9),* Hubbard, R., & Lindsay, R. M. From significant differences to significant sameness: Proposing a paradigm shift in business research. 1377–1388, 2013, with permission from Elsevier.

integrity continues to be questioned (Cumming, 2014), particularly that related to biased publication practices, selective data analyses, and absent replication. NHST reliance is a critical factor influencing research integrity. These practices foster persistence of false conclusions.

What do investigators interested in nursing education research need to do as they undertake the conduct and reporting of research? A least five significant practices warrant being undertaken: Nurse scientists need to have a better understanding of the limitations of NHST, as well as what p values connote; increase their use and reporting of confidence intervals (CIs); include discussion of effect size when reporting data; and undertake more replication. Each is discussed in the following sections.

Limitations of Null Hypothesis Significance Testing

Most investigators, including this author, would argue they are well educated about NHST and how to interpret p values. Unfortunately, experts are vocal in their efforts to dispel this assumption (Cumming, 2012, 2014; Kline, 2013; Hubbard, 2016; Reinhart, 2015). Readers are encouraged to review the aforementioned references for an in-depth discussion. For now, the following are offered for clarity. Cumming (2012) states that "[t]he p value is the probability of getting our observed results, or a more extreme result, if the null hypothesis is true" (p. 27). Note that this definition refers to the probability of obtaining observed results, not to the probability that the null hypothesis is true (Cumming, 2012). Nor does the p value indicate that "results are due to chance" (Cumming, 2012, p. 28), a statement found in some statistics textbooks. Consider the following statements: "The probability of getting certain results if the null is true" versus "The probability that the null is true if we've obtained certain results" (Cumming, 2012, p. 27). Although investigators want the p value to reflect the latter quotation, it is the former quotation that conveys the true meaning associated with a p value. Moreover, Cumming cautions investigators "not to take statistical nonsignificance (the null is not rejected) as evidence of a zero effect (the null is true)" (p. 29). He also urges investigators to guard against treating nonsignificant findings as no findings. In other words, nonsignificant differences are not the same as no difference.

What does this mean for investigators investigating research questions relevant to nursing education? A first step for nurse scientists is to review how they have typically interpreted the p value in light of the preceding discussion. Then they can consider alternative approaches to presenting information to enhance understanding of their findings so that they are meaningful to a range of readers. Two YouTube videos are particularly helpful when reviewing the meaning of p values:

▶ Cumming, G. *Intro Statistics 9: Dance of the p Values* (a great video explaining the limitations of p value): https://www.youtube.com/watch?v=5OL1RqHrZQ8

▶ Kiss, A. *Learn statistics: The correct definition of the p-value:* https://www.youtube.com/watch?v=oM_I6ilwx0Q

Increase the Use of Confidence Intervals

CIs are offered as one practice that experts believe helps to address the significant difference paradigm discussed earlier in this section (Cumming, 2012; Hubbard, 2016; Kline, 2013; Reinhart, 2015). Cumming and Finch (2005) highlight four major advantages of CIs: They (a) provide point and interval estimates in measurement units that are understandable, (b) underscore a link to p values and the NHST, (c) "[h]elp combine evidence over experiments" (p. 171) (think replication), and (d) provide precision or variability information.

CIs have become an important piece of information to include when presenting results. In fact, the American Psychological Association (APA) (2010) strongly recommends the use of CIs, as they "combine information on location and precision and can often be directly used to infer significance levels" (p. 34). Yet a cursory review of the major papers published in the *Journal of Nursing Education* and *Nursing Education Perspectives* during 2014 and 2015 revealed that few authors reported CIs when presenting results for which CIs would be appropriate. Such a finding is made even more disturbing given that both of these journals indicate that authors should follow APA guidelines for publication.

CIs are key to being able to see how individual study results compare to each other. They play a key role in replication of studies, as replication may produce equally significant *p* values but very disparate CIs, raising questions about what is known about a particular phenomenon. Fortunately, Cumming (2012) has developed software that helps explicate key concepts associated with CIs (available at http://erin.sfn.org/resources/2012/04/16/exploratory-software-for-confidence-intervals-comma-esci?su=q/[,]/t//s//a//e//r//g//dr/0/cp/4/rsp/50/sm/1/sc/0).

Determine the Effect Size

Nurse scientists are familiar with discussions about effect size, as effect size is a critical element, among several others, when determining sample size. In essence, *effect size* "is the main finding in quantitative research" (Sullivan & Feinn, 2012, p. 279). Absolute effect sizes, such as the calculated difference between group means, are more useful when variables have intrinsic meaning. For example, an absolute effect size would be used when reporting results using grade point average as the variable of interest. When variables cannot be directly compared, as assessment instruments have varied, "standardized measures of effect, which are calculated to transform the effect to an easily understood scale" (Sullivan & Feinn, 2012, p. 279), can be employed. Nurse scientists are familiar with such effect size indices as Cohen's *d,* odds ratio, and relative risk, which are used when examining between group differences; measures of association effect size indices include Pearson's *r* correlation and r^2 coefficient of determination (Sullivan & Feinn, 2012). Yet rarely are these indices reported and interpreted in publications addressing research relevant to nursing education. Moreover, effect sizes should be determined based on how best to answer relevant disciplinary questions (Cumming, 2014). Finally, Cumming (2012) reminds readers that a "*p* value is *not* an ES [effect size]" (p. 15). If the science of nursing education is to advance, then investigators addressing nursing education will need to incorporate this behavior into their research practice when conducting quantitative research.

Increase the Use of Replication

Replication is the hallmark of science. Furthermore, replication of original results guards against the presence of specious findings (Hubbard, 2016). Indeed, if the science of nursing education is to be advanced, investigators must undertake replication of their studies. Nursing education literature is replete with one-shot studies, few have been replicated, and many undertaken as large studies are disseminated as pilot studies due to methodological issues such as small sample sizes. Embracing a significant sameness paradigm fosters the use of replication, as does embracing the practice of asking oneself the following question when reading the results of a study: "I wonder whether similar results would occur if the study were repeated?" This type of question conveys an investigator's appreciation of the larger perspective relative to their area of research. Cumming (2014) urges investigators to use meta-analytic thinking—one study builds on prior work that then informs future work.

Authors differentiate between types of replication (Drotar, 2010), as well as among associated terms such as *reproducibility* (Asendorpf et al., 2013). Although there is overlap, several perspectives are discussed in greater detail. Drotar (2010) differentiates between internal and external replication. Internal replication occurs when a sample from an existing dataset is randomly selected. This strategy, termed *cross-validation,* results in performing the identical analyses as were performed on the original sample. Select statistical procedures, such as bootstrapping, can assist investigators with the type of replication. Drotar does not indicate who conducts the replication. Asendorpf et al. (2013), on the other hand, consider this type of replication consistent with reproducibility and make explicit that someone other than the original investigator obtains the same statistical and estimate results using the same data and methodology.

Drotar (2010) offers that eternal replication occurs when data are collected from new samples at different times. Interestingly, Asendorpf et al. (2013) consider this reflective of replicability. Moreover, critical to their perspective is that sampling is comprehensive in nature and extends beyond participants.

Irrespective of definition, certain characteristics are key to replication: where data are obtained (sample), how data are obtained (measures), and how data are analyzed. These characteristics, originally described by Tsang and Kwan (1999), are presented in Table 7.2. Additional considerations include timeliness of replication efforts (i.e., stipulating how long after the original work does replication occur); availability of data (how willing is the original investigator to share the data?); insufficient power; and of critical importance, determining whether the original work is worthy of replication. Notwithstanding these considerations, it is incumbent on investigators interested in advancing the science of nursing education to undertake efforts to replicate their own research efforts, as well as those of other investigators. Only then will investigators advance the science of nursing education—an advancement that is sorely needed.

TABLE 7.2

A Typology of Replication

Source of Data	Same Measurement and Analysis	Different Measurement and/or Analysis
Same data set	Checking of analysis	Reanalysis of the data
Same population	Exact replication	Conceptual extension
Different population	Empirical generalizations	Generalizations and extensions

SOURCE: Tsang, E. W. K., & Kwan, K. M. (1999). Replication and theory development in organizational science: A critical realist perspective. *Academy of Management Review, 24,* 759–790.

Acknowledging the Role of Qualitative Research in Statistical Cognition Research

Interestingly, Kalinowski, Lai, Fidler, and Cumming (2010) have argued that including qualitative research enhances understanding of "cognitive processes, representations, and activities involved in acquiring and using statistical knowledge" (p. 22). Not only does qualitative research enhance the description of the phenomenon under investigation, it also can provide insight about new directions for exploration. This best practice calls for the use of more multimethod approaches with all aspects of research, particularly those related to data analysis and interpretation. Investigators may wish to consider this practice when undertaking future research efforts in nursing education.

Developing Expertise in Big Data Processes

No discussion of future data collection, analysis, and interpretation would be complete without mention of the role that Big Data now plays in generating knowledge. *Big Data* is a term used to describe a "dataset that is too large to easily manipulate and manage" (Austin & Kusumoto, 2016, para 2). Key elements of Big Data are volume, variety, and velocity (Austin & Kusumoto, 2016; Roski, Bo-Linn, & Andrews, 2014). Volume—that is, the amount of data generated annually—"is projected to double every 2 years" (Austin & Kusumoto, 2016, para 4). There is more variety in the data generated currently. Text messages, streaming video, and Fitbit™ recordings are all forms of data that are less structured, yet analyzing them could provide meaningful information. Data are now generated in real time, calling for rapid processing solutions that address the need for decreased time required for analysis.

One approach to data analysis is the use of machine learning. This approach, "also known as pattern recognition, represents a range of techniques used to analyze big data by identifying patterns of interaction among variables" (Passos, Mwangi, & Kapczinski, 2016, p. 13). This approach, unlike traditional statistical methods that consider group results, allows for examination of outcomes at the individual level.

The term *Big Data* is often associated with health care, as analyzing large datasets can be the impetus for "improving health outcomes while lowering costs" (Roski et al., 2014, p. 1115). Nurse faculty, although familiar with discussions occurring relative to information contained in electronic health records, may question the relevance of Big Data to their practice. However, the Robert Wood Johnson Foundation recently awarded a grant to several investigators to develop a national network to collect appropriate data from schools of nursing (http://www.rwjf.org/en/library/grants/2015/02/developing-a-national-research-network-to-generate-evidence-for-.html). The network, called the *National Nursing Education Research Network* (NNERN), is an example of what will be a huge dataset amenable to Big Data analysis techniques. If investigators are to take advantage of these resources, they will need to develop an understanding and expertise in analyzing Big Data.

CONCLUSIONS AND IMPLICATIONS

Applying best practices to manage, analyze, and interpret data exist, yet evidence indicates that investigators have not adhered to them consistently. Many best practices highlighted in this chapter reflect efforts to counter QRPs. Moreover, future efforts have been explicated. Armed with this information, investigators addressing relevant nursing education research questions can contribute to building a more robust body of nursing education knowledge.

References

American Psychological Association. (2010). *Publication manual of the American Psychological Association* (6th ed.). Washington, DC: Author.

Asendorpf, J. B., Conner, M., De Fruyt, F., De Houwer, J., Denissen, J. J. A., Fiedler, K., et al. (2013). Recommendations for increasing replicability in psychology. *European Journal of Personality, 27*, 108–119. doi:10.1002/per.1919

Austin, C., & Kusumoto, F. (2016). The application of Big Data in medicine: Current implications and future directions. *Journal of Interventional Cardiac Electrophysiology.* Published online January 27, 2016. doi:10.1007/s10840-016-0104-y

Cumming, G. (2012). *Understanding the new statistics: Effect sizes, confidence intervals, and meta-analysis.* New York: Routledge.

Cumming, G. (2014). The new statistics: Why and how. *Psychological Science, 25*(1), 7–29. doi:10.1177/00956797613504966

Cumming, G., & Finch, S. (2005). Inference by eye: Confidence intervals and how to read pictures of data. *American Psychologist, 60*, 170–180. doi:10.1037/0003-006X.60.2.170

Drotar, D. (2010). Editorial: A call for replications of research in pediatric psychology and guidance for authors. *Journal of Pediatric Psychology, 35*, 801–805. doi:10.1093/jpepsy/jsq049

Fanelli, D. (2009). How many scientists fabricate and falsify research? A systematic review and meta-analysis of survey data. *PLoS ONE, 4*(5), e5738. doi:10.1371/journal.pone.0005738

Fierz, K., Gennaro, S., Dierickx, K., Van Achterberg, T., Morin, K. H., De Geest, S., et al. (2014). Scientific misconduct: Also an issue in nursing science? *Journal of Nursing Scholarship, 46*, 271–280. doi:10.1111/jnu.12082

Hayat, J. H., Higgins, M., Schwartz, T. A., & Staggs, V. S. (2015). Statistical challenges in nursing education and research: An expert panel consensus. *Nurse Educator, 40*(1), 21–25. doi:10.1097/NNE.0000000000000080

Hayat, M. J., Schmiege, S. J., & Cook, P. F. (2014). Perspectives on statistics education: Observations from statistical consulting in an academic nursing environment. *Journal of Nursing Education, 53*, 185–191. doi:10.3928/0148434-20140321-01

Horner, J., & Minifie, F. D. (2011). Research ethics II: Mentoring, collaboration, peer review, and data management and ownership. *Journal of Speech, Language, and Hearing Research, 54*, S320–S345. doi:10.1044/1092-4388(2010/09-0264)

Hubbard, R. (2016). *Corrupt research: The case of reconceptualizing empirical management and social science.* Thousand Oaks, CA: Sage.

Ironside, P. M., & Spurlock, D. R. (2014). Editorial: Getting serious about building nursing education science. *Journal of Nursing Education, 53*, 667–669. doi:10.3928/01484834-20141118-10

Jeličić, H., Phelps, E., & Lerner, R. M. (2009). Use of missing data methods in longitudinal studies: The persistence of bad practices in developmental psychology. *Developmental Psychology, 45*, 1195–1199. doi:10.1037/a00115665

John, L. K., Loewenstein, G., & Prelec, D. (2012). Measuring the prevalence of questionable research practices with incentives for truth telling. *Psychological Science, 23*, 524–532. doi:10.1117/0956797611430953

Kalichman, M., Sweet, M., & Plemmons, D. (2014). Standards of scientific conduct: Are there any? *Science and Engineering Ethics, 20*, 885–896. doi:10.1007/s11948-013-9500-1

Kalichman, M., Sweet, M., & Plemmons, D. (2015). Standards of scientific conduct: Disciplinary differences. *Science and Engineering Ethics, 20*, 885–896. doi:10.1007/s11948-014-9594-0

Kalinowski, P., Lai, J., Fidler, F., & Cumming, G. (2010). Qualitative research: An essential part of statistical cognition research. *Statistics Education Research Journal, 9*(2), 22–34.

Kerr, N. L. (1998). HARKing: Hypothesizing after the results are known. *Personality and Social Psychology Review, 2*, 197–217.

Kline, R. B. (2013). *Beyond significance testing: Statistics reform in the behavioral sciences* (2nd ed.). Washington, DC: American Psychological Association.

Laine, C., Goodman, S. N., Griswold, M. E., & Sox, H. C. (2007). Reproducible research: Moving toward research that public can really trust. *Annals of Internal Medicine, 146*, 450–453.

Macrina, F. L. (Ed.). (2014). Scientific record keeping. In *Scientific integrity. Text and cases in responsible conduct of research* (4th ed., pp. 329–359). Washington, DC: ASM Press.

Marco, C. A., & Larkin, G. L. (2000). Research ethics: Ethical issues of data reporting and the quest for authenticity. *Academic Emergency Medicine, 7*, 691–694.

Marshall, C., & Rossman, G. B. (2016). *Designing qualitative research* (6th ed.). Los Angeles: Sage.

Miles, M. B., Huberman, A. M., & Saldaña, J. (2014). *Qualitative data analysis: A methods sourcebook* (3rd ed.). Los Angeles: Sage.

Minkler, M. (2005). Community-based research partnerships: Challenges and opportunities. *Journal of Urban Health: Bulletin of the New York Academy of Medicine, 82*(2, Suppl. 3), ii3–ii12. doi:10.1093/jurban/jti034

Morin, K. H. (2013). Value of a pilot study. *Journal of Nursing Education, 52*, 547–548. doi:10.3928/01484834-20130920-10

Morin, K. H. (2014). Nursing education: The past, present and future. *Journal of Health Specialties, 2*(4), 6–11. doi:10.4103/1658-600X.142781

Passos, I. C., Mwangi, B., & Kapczinski, F. (2016). Comment: Big Data analytics and machine learning: 2015 and beyond. *Lancet Psychiatry 3*, 13–15. doi:10.1016/S2215-0366(15)00549-0

Reinhart, A. (2015). *Statistics done wrong.* San Francisco: No Starch Press.

Roski, J., Bo-Linn, G. W., & Andrews, T. A. (2014). Creating value in health care through Big Data: Opportunities and policy implications. *Health Affairs, 33*, 1115–1122. doi:10.1377/hlthaff.2014.0147

Sandelowski, M. (2010). What's in a name? Qualitative description revisited. *Research in Nursing and Health, 33*, 77–84. doi:10.1002/nur.20362

Scheier, A. A., Wilson, K., & Resnik, D. (2006). Academic research record-keeping: Best practices for individuals, group leaders, and institutions. *Academic Medicine, 81*, 42–47.

Sijtsma, K. (2015). Playing with data—or how to discourage questionable research practices and stimulate researchers to do things right. *Psychometrika, 81*(1), 1–15.

Spellman, B. A. (2013). Open peer commentary: There is no such thing as replication, but we should do it anyway. *European Journal of Personality, 27*, 120–144. doi:10.1002/per.1920

Steneck, N. H. (2007). *ORI: Introduction to the responsible conduct of research.* Washington, DC: U.S. Department of Health and Human Services. USBN: 976-0-16-072285-1

St. Pierre Schneider, B., Nicholas, J., & Kumus, J. (2013). Comparison of methodologic quality and study/report characteristics between quantitative clinical nursing and nursing education research articles. *Nursing Education Perspectives, 34*, 292–297. doi:10.5480/1536-5026-34.5.292

Strasser, C., Cook, R., Michener, W., & Buddin, A. (n.d.). Primer on data management: What you always wanted to know. *DataONE Best Practice Primer.* Available at https://www.dataone.org

Sullivan, G. M., & Feinn, R. (2012). Using effect size—or why the P value is not enough. *Journal of Graduate Medical Education, 4*, 279–282. doi:10.4300/JGME-D-12-00156.1

Tong, A., Sainsbury, P., & Craig, J. (2007). Consolidated criteria for reporting qualitative research (COREQ): A 32-item checklist for interviews and focus groups. *International Journal for Quality in Health Care, 19*, 349–357. doi:10.1093/intqhc/mzm042

Tsang, E. W. K., & Kwan, K. M. (1999). Replication and theory development in organizational science: A critical realist perspective. *Academy of Management Review, 24*, 759–790.

Ulrich, C. M., Wallen, G. R., Cui, N., Chittmans, J., Sweet, M., & Plemmons, D. (2015). Establishing good collaborative research practices in the responsible conduct of research in nursing science. *Nursing Outlook, 63*, 171–180. doi:10.1016/j.oulook.2014.10.007

Valiga, T. M., & Ironside, P. M. (2012). Guest editorial: Crafting a national agenda for nursing education research. *Journal of Nursing Education, 51*, 3–4. doi:10.3928/0148434-20111213-01

8

Evidence-Based Teaching: Moving Evidence into Practice

Teresa Shellenbarger, PhD, RN, CNE, ANEF

Recent reports about nursing and health care have forced nursing faculty to examine the approaches used to prepare nurses for practice. Benner, Sutphen, Leonard, and Day (2009), in their book *Educating Nurses: A Call for Radical Transformation,* suggest a need for profound changes in nursing education and propose one essential approach that requires a greater focus on the scholarship of teaching and learning. The 3-year follow-up progress report of this study suggests that some schools are responding to this call with curriculum and pedagogy changes, but further work is needed (Benner, 2013). Similarly, the National League for Nursing (NLN) (2012) encouraged change in nursing education and advocated for advancing evidence-based teaching. This chapter discusses how faculty can apply nursing education research to enhance teaching practice. The chapter begins by discussing how investigators can disseminate research findings through presentations and publications. Once this evidence is shared publically, faculty begin the challenging process of changing the educational culture and building nursing education on sound evidence-based practice. The chapter continues with an examination of the integration of research evidence into educational practices, and it concludes with a discussion about the influence of nursing education research on policy.

DISSEMINATION OF RESEARCH ABOUT TEACHING PRACTICE

At the completion of a research study, investigators must disseminate their work to advance knowledge. Dissemination involves the active and planned spread of information—in this case, nursing education research. Sharing research findings with others can be helpful for faculty and nursing leaders who will use this information to make decisions about teaching and learning practices, evaluation of students, curriculum modifications, or enhancements of nursing education. Research findings also provide the foundation for future studies and aid in the identification of the knowledge gaps that remain. However, for nursing education research to be truly helpful to others, it must be shared publicly and customized for the intended users. Nursing education investigators have two primary avenues for dissemination. Research can be shared through presentations and publications. The following portion of this chapter will discuss important considerations when disseminating research.

Presentations

Many investigators present their nursing education research findings at scholarly conferences. Presentations allow for rapid dissemination of the study findings; however, investigators will want to consider a variety of factors when determining the appropriate format and forum for presentation. One aspect for investigators to consider involves the focus of the conference. Some conferences, such as the National League for Nursing (NLN)/Sigma Theta Tau International (STTI) Nursing Education Research Conference, are devoted exclusively to the reporting of research studies in nursing education. Presentations made at conferences that focus solely on nursing education are shared with attendees who clearly have an interest in nursing educational research. Other research conferences, such as the Sigma Theta Tau International Biennium, will include research reports in various clinical and educational areas, so attendees of these conferences may have an interest in broad research topics and not just nursing education research. A third type of conference, such as the NLN Education Summit, may have non-research-based presentations occurring concurrently with nursing education research presentations. Attendees at such conferences may have varying backgrounds, knowledge, and interest in educational research.

Another aspect for investigators to consider when choosing a venue for sharing their educational research involves the scope of the conference. Some conferences may just draw audiences from local or regional areas. Some investigators might consider a conference with a larger scope and will want to consider conferences that draw participants from a much wider geographic area, such as national conferences or even international conferences. Investigators will want to carefully consider the most appropriate audience for sharing their findings and select the best match. Box 8.1 provides a variety of organizations that typically host conferences providing opportunities to present nursing education research and can help faculty when making dissemination decisions.

Investigators will want to consider the estimated number of conference attendees and the size of the anticipated audience in attendance for the presentation, as this will influence how many people may hear the presentation and learn about the study,

---

BOX 8.1

Nursing Conferences That Include Nursing Education Research

NLN/STTI Nursing Education Research Conference
STTI Research Congress
International Nursing Education Conference (NETNEP)
NLN Education Summit
STTI Biennial Convention
American Association of Colleges of Nursing Education Conferences
Conferences sponsored by publishing companies or other businesses involved with nursing education
Regional Research conferences (Eastern Nursing Research Society, Southern Nursing Research Society,
    Midwest Nursing Research Society, Western Institute of Nursing)
Conferences sponsored by educational organizations
Local or regional STTI chapter events

thereby impacting the dissemination of the results. In addition, investigators will want to consider the conference location and the attendees participating in the conference. International conferences will enable the investigator to share findings with a global audience, whereas a regional conference will probably reach a much smaller geographic audience. Studies that have data collection from multiple sites that use large national or international representative samples, or investigate nursing education topics impacting educators and students in many locations, might be best suited for national or international conferences. Studies that are smaller in scope, have sampling limitations that impact generalizability, are based on pilot studies, or investigate indigenous educational issues may be better suited for regional or local conferences.

Finally, investigators will want to consider the format of the presentation when making dissemination decisions. Many conferences offer the option to present either in a poster or oral presentation format. Poster presentations provide a self-paced, informal, intimate opportunity to share study information in a visual display, either on poster boards or electronically. Conference attendees browse displayed posters and engage in informal discussions with the poster presenters. Posters are also appropriate for preliminary findings or pilot study reports. Oral presentations usually provide a more formal opportunity to share completed study findings via a narrative session to a larger audience. These oral presentations typically report completed research projects.

Investigators should watch for a call for abstracts announcing the solicitation of research presentations. Potential presenters should carefully follow the submission guidelines. Submissions should include a clear, concise, and cohesive summary of the project. The abstract submission should reflect the theme or focus of the conference, as well as align with the anticipated audience. Investigators will also want to consider the timing of the conference and submission date of the abstract. Some conferences have a rapid review and short time between the call for abstracts and the conference, thus allowing investigators to rapidly disseminate their findings. Other conferences have a longer delay between the announced call for abstracts and presentation time. In this case, investigators may have to wait many months before their findings can be shared at those conferences, thus prolonging the time for dissemination. Nursing education investigators should consider these factors when planning the best presentation for their work so that knowledge is shared at the right time with the right people.

Publications

To share nursing education research findings with other faculty, investigators will also want to publish their work. Typically, publication of nursing education research involves journal articles that focus on specific teaching and learning strategies. Occasionally, some nursing education research will be published as part of a book, such as the research reported in the book *Educating Nurses: A Call for Radical Transformation* (Benner et al., 2009).

There are a series of steps that nurse investigators take when attempting to publish their nursing education research in nursing or related journals. The first step involves identifying the appropriate journal to target for publication. Just like conferences, journals may focus specifically on nursing education topics, others might focus on clinical practice topics, and some journals may include a combination of topics. Clinically focused journals may occasionally publish education articles, especially if it impacts practice issues. Table 8.1

TABLE 8.1

Journals That Publish Nursing Education Research

Journal Name	Website	Focus
International Journal of Nursing Education Scholarship	http://www.degruyter.com/view/j/ijnes	Publishes research and scholarship in nursing education.
Journal for Nurses in Staff Development	http://www.researchgate.net/journal/1098-7886_Journal_for_Nurses_in_Staff_Development-JNSD	Articles focus on issues that impact staff development.
Journal of Continuing Education in Nursing	http://www.healio.com/nursing/journals/jcen	Publishes articles directed toward continuing education and staff development professionals, nurse administrators, and nursing faculty in all health care settings.
Journal of Nursing Education	http://www.healio.com/nursing/journals/jne	Publishes research and other scholarly works involving and influencing nursing education. Focuses on aspects of nursing education related to undergraduate and graduate nursing programs.
Journal of Professional Nursing	http://www.professionalnursing.org	Focuses on baccalaureate- and higher-degree nursing education, educational research, and policy related to education.
Nurse Education Today	http://www.nurseeducationtoday.com	Publishes original research, review, and debate in the discussion of nursing. Publishes papers that contribute to the advancement of educational theory and pedagogy that support evidence-based practice worldwide.
Nurse Educator	http://journals.lww.com/nurseeducatoronline/pages/default.aspx	Provides practical information and research related to nursing education.
Nursing Education in Practice	http://www.journals.elsevier.com/nurse-education-in-practice	Disseminates evidence about educational practice in clinical or university settings.
Nursing Education Perspectives	http://www.nln.org/newsroom/newsletters-and-journal/nursing-education-perspectives-journal	Focuses on nursing education research with preference given to large-scale national studies or those that go beyond an exploratory nature.
Teaching and Learning in Nursing	http://www.jtln.org	Focuses on the advancement of associate-degree nursing education and practice.

*Data not reported.
NA, not applicable.
(From NAHRS Research Committee Journal Project Team, 2012; Northam et al., 2014.)

No. per Year	Research (%)	Acceptance Rate (%)	Time to Review	Acceptance to Publication Print/Online	Format
1/year; updated continuously	*	*	*	*	Online
6	31.03	*	*	*	Print/online
12	29.56	41	8 weeks	16/16 weeks	Print/online
12	47.32	18–20	4 weeks	*	Print/online
6	51.45	27	7 weeks	10/10 weeks	Print/online
12	73.39	*	*	*	Print/online
6	16.49	18	2 weeks	36 weeks/NA	Print/online
4	66.22	59	12 weeks	24–36/ 24 weeks	Print/online
6	24.95	22	14 weeks	71/71 weeks	Print and online for NLN members
4	*	50	16 weeks	*	Print/online

provides a listing of some journals that frequently publish nursing education topics. The table also provides some additional information about each journal, including frequency of publication, focus of the journal, and format. As can be seen in the table, some of these nursing journals are primarily research based. Others may contain a mix of research and non-research-based topics, such as anecdotal, informational, or opinion pieces.

Investigators will want to explore potential journals and evaluate the best fit for the dissemination of their study. They may want to consider the audience the journal reaches (international or national focus, faculty or clinician), format of the journal (traditional print, online, and/or free digital open access), aim and scope of the journal, and circulation of the journal. The investigator will want to select a target publication that aligns with the topic and potential reader interest. There are additional factors that the investigator will want to consider. One factor involves how long it takes to get the work published in a particular journal. Northam, Greer, Rath, and Toone (2014) conducted a study of 61 nursing journals and reported that nursing journals publish between 1 and 18 times per year, but the average number of issues is 6 per year. Frequency of publication may impact the time it takes to get the work in press and disseminated to readers. This is an important consideration, as timely dissemination is critical for new or cutting-edge topics that may impact educational practices.

Another factor impacting publication time is the review process. On average, acceptance notification occurs in about 8 weeks, but it can vary from a few weeks to as many as 18 weeks (Northam et al., 2014). Investigators may then face a waiting period until the work is publically available to readers, which also varies by journal. With the advent of open access formats and online journals, many articles are now available for viewing much sooner than in the past with traditional print journals. Investigators wanting to publish time-sensitive topics should consider these factors when deciding the best journal fit.

Investigators should also think about the discoverability of the article and will want readers to be able to search and locate the article through traditional search mechanisms, such as electronic databases like the Cumulative Index to Nursing and Allied Health Literature (CINAHL®). Select journals provide indexing in databases that readers will typically use, and select keywords and titles that will aid in identification and retrieval of the work. Finally, investigators may consider acceptance rates of the journal, which can vary from as low as 10 percent to greater than 90 percent (Northam et al., 2014). Keep in mind that these rates fluctuate. Nursing education journal statistics reported in Table 8.1 are gathered from the Nursing and Allied Health Resources Section (NAHRS) of the Medical Library Association's selected list of nursing journals (Nursing and Allied Health Resources Section Research Committee Journal Project Team, 2012) and represent a snapshot of data during the reported period. Some journals do not have acceptance rates reported in the table, as this information was not available for review. Regardless, these rates should not be the sole determinant for journal selection, as there are multiple explanations for these acceptance rates. Nursing education investigators should consider all of these factors when selecting the best choice for publication of their work.

Dissemination Structure

Once the investigator has selected a conference or journal for dissemination, he or she will need to obtain the submission guidelines and follow the instructions provided. Most research, particularly quantitative research reports, will follow the IMRaD format for reporting. IMRaD is an acronym that represents the major headings of a research report, including the introduction, methods, results, and discussion. Key components that should be included in each of the sections when reporting education research will be discussed in the following section.

The introduction provides important background information and helps to establish the need for the study. It explains why this was a worthy topic for investigation and the problem faced in nursing education. The introduction also includes the research questions and the purpose of the study. The theoretical framework guiding the study may be part of the introduction as well. Including information about the theory used provides an organizing structure to the research and explains the conceptual connections between phenomena. Many investigators will include a selective review of key literature as part of the background of the study. This literature provides a synthesis of critical knowledge about the topic. Finally, the introduction identifies the knowledge gaps that remain about a topic, thus serving as a justification for the study (Mertler & Charles, 2015).

The next section involves the methods or procedures of the study. The investigator provides a step-by-step explanation of the methods of data collection, the sampling, and the analysis of the data. Research reports should also include a description of how subjects' rights were protected and an indication of review by an institutional review board. The data collection tools should be described and include an overview of the format, scoring, and use of the tools. Descriptions of the reliability and validity of the measures are also usually reported for quantitative studies. Qualitative studies should describe the methods used to establish quality, such as measures taken to ensure confirmability, trustworthiness, auditability, credibility, dependability, and transferability (Oermann & Hays, 2015). Investigators should provide information about the population under investigation and how subjects were recruited and selected, as well as inclusion and exclusion criteria for the sample (International Committee of Medical Journal Editors, 2011). An explanation of the adequacy of the sample size is also needed. These sampling components are important to allow readers to assess generalizability. The methods section typically ends with a description of the data analysis.

The results of the study will follow the methods section. Investigators should provide an informative narrative description of the findings that answer the study questions. Typically, investigators report the sample demographics and descriptive statistics. Tables and figures may be helpful. Inferential statistics typically follow in a quantitative study. Investigators should report the statistical test or method of analysis used, verification that the data conformed to statistical test assumptions, the specific findings, and the level of statistical significance. The findings should be presented with enough detail to verify reported results and incorporate this work in future studies or for replication (Glasziou et al., 2014; Lang & Altman, 2014). For qualitative studies, investigators report methods of data analysis, emergent findings, and narrative exemplars, quotes, or statements that describe the phenomenon of interest (Oermann & Hays, 2015).

The investigator concludes with a discussion that interprets the data and explains their meaning. This section also includes conclusions and a discussion about how the findings relate to nursing education. Usually, investigators provide recommendations for how to apply the findings to nursing education and offer suggestions for further research. This is particularly helpful for advancing evidence-based teaching practice (EBTP), as it provides suggestions for use. It helps to explain how the findings can be used in education and where gaps still remain. It can also provide ideas for the development of an ongoing research trajectory about a nursing education topic that will further enhance knowledge about the topic. All studies will have some limitations, and these potential problems are addressed in the discussion section. This reporting format ensures that all components of the study are reported in a uniform manner while also providing enough information to assess relevance and applicability in nursing education.

CHANGING CULTURE AND UNDERSTANDING ABOUT EVIDENCE-BASED TEACHING PRACTICE

Sharing nursing education research through presentations and publications is an important step in advancing EBTP, as the dissemination of this research knowledge is shared with nursing audiences. However, it does not ensure the use of findings in nursing education practice. The culture or environment of the educational workplace can either help or hinder the utilization and translation of evidence into teaching practice. The literature is replete with discussions about barriers and facilitators of evidence-based nursing practice in a clinical setting (Gale & Schaffer, 2009; Melnyk, Fineout-Overholt, Gallagher-Ford, & Kaplan, 2012). Many of these same barriers exist in nursing education and may slow the use of research findings in education. Faculty need to consider the individual and organizational barriers faced in implementing EBTP and strategize approaches to minimize them. The following section discusses the barriers that faculty may face and offers suggestions to promote application of findings into teaching practice.

Faculty report a variety of personal barriers that impact the use of research in nursing education. Common barriers include demanding workloads and insufficient time to devote to reading the research literature (Patterson & Klein, 2012). They may also have limited access to research reports. Additionally, many nursing faculty, particularly those with clinical backgrounds, enter academia without extensive formal educational preparation and research course work. Their educational preparation may only provide the basic fundamentals needed for critiquing research. Or they may not have recent practice critiquing research or sufficient expertise to critique nursing education research and make decisions about use in practice.

There are institutional barriers that may hamper the use of evidence in nursing education. Having a lack of supportive leaders and mentors, as well as a lack of organizational commitment to EBTP, can also pose barriers (Dang & White, 2012; Hauck, Wisett, & Kuric, 2012; Melnyk et al., 2012). Nursing faculty proposing alternative approaches to traditional educational practice may face resistance when making educational changes, even when these changes are supported by the evidence.

Despite facing some of these same barriers in clinical practice settings, nurses are making progress in the implementation of evidence-based care, and this suggests that faculty can overcome implementation barriers as well. The literature discussing

TABLE 8.2	
Evidence-Based Teaching Practice Goals and Strategies	
Goals	**Strategies**
Establish support for EBTP initiatives.	Library resources (databases, electronic journals) Budgetary support for EBTP activities Faculty workload assignment
Develop EBTP mentors who can assist and guide the change process.	Identify mentors Train mentors Support mentors Recognize and reward mentors
Develop a critical mass of EBTP champions.	Identify early adopters of EBTP Role model EBTP Reward and recognize EBTP champions
Discuss EBTP with colleagues and administrators.	Journal clubs EBTP workshops Faculty meetings Online learning modules
Facilitate dissemination of EBTP and outcomes.	Faculty recognition Policy development Presentations Publications
Establish and measure outcomes.	Develop data collection plans Collect data to determine effectiveness of changes

evidence-based nursing practice in clinical settings provides some helpful suggestions that can be applied to nursing education to overcome some of the personal and environmental barriers faced. Organizational leaders possess power and influence, and through their actions they can model the culture change needed for acceptance of EBTP. They can encourage, support, recognize, and reward nursing faculty who are making changes based on the research evidence. Identifying EBTP goals and implementation strategies that can be used by nursing faculty may also assist in EBTP enculturation. Hauck et al. (2012) report on a strategic plan used to address evidence-based practice enculturation in a hospital setting. This plan can be adapted for use with EBTP planning in education. Suggested goals and strategies are outlined in Table 8.2. Goals can focus on establishing support for EBTP, developing EBTP mentors, creating a critical mass of EBTP champions, and/or discussing EBTP with others. Gaining leadership support, facilitating dissemination, and implementing strategies to measure outcomes are also important parts of the plan. Shifts in the cultural beliefs will take time when aided by ongoing support from campus leaders (Ginsberg & Bernstein, 2011).

A variety of factors can help to create an environment supportive of EBTP. To effectively use research in nursing education, faculty must have access to adequate resources. They need to be able to search a variety of databases to identify appropriate references. Many nursing faculty will use CINAHL® for literature searches, but they also need access to other useful databases, such as ERIC®, ProQuest®, SocINDEX®, and PsycINFO®, that may contain relevant education topics. Reference librarians can provide useful guidance when searching databases and offer suggestions for key search terms or for improving search results and provide additional human resources to support EBTP (Hauck et al., 2012). Once citations are identified through searches, faculty need to gain access to journals and the research articles. Key individuals within the institution can help to address access problems (Kalb, O'Conner-Von, Brockway, Rierson, & Sendelbach, 2015). Institutional leaders may need to champion EBTP and advocate to reduce access and implementation barriers.

Mentors can guide faculty who are new to using EBTP, and they can assist with searching, critiquing, and planning the use of research findings into teaching activities. Some faculty may need assistance in the translation of research findings into educational practices and will benefit from faculty development initiatives. Planning informative programs related to EBTP topics will help to ensure a critical mass of faculty who have the knowledge, skills, and know-how to incorporate evidence into teaching practices. Additionally, influential institutional leaders can assist in ensuring that EBTP is an important component of faculty performance evaluation processes such as tenure and promotion.

One strategy to advance research use that is reported in the nursing literature identifies journal clubs as an approach to engaging staff with evidence-based activities. Journal clubs have been effectively used in clinical practice to provide a relaxed, welcoming, and supportive atmosphere to discuss nursing research (Lachance, 2014). Journal clubs might also benefit faculty wishing to advance EBTP. Including interdisciplinary faculty, such as those with a background and interest in teaching and higher education, can contribute valuable insight into the discussions about educational research reports. Meeting and networking with faculty colleagues across the campus to discuss education-focused research will enhance critical appraisal skills, promote team building and collaboration, and provide an opportunity to discuss teaching practices. Engaging in a dialogue about research with a community of faculty colleagues can help to build support, empower faculty, and accelerate improvements, and may lead to policy reform.

There are obstacles that faculty may encounter when beginning discussions with nursing and campus colleagues; however, some simple strategies may address these problems. Since time limitations are a major barrier to EBTP, there are some things that might improve time efficiency. Sharing research articles with faculty colleagues, particularly with the use of electronic delivery, will decrease the burden of searching, locating, and retrieving research articles. Each faculty member could select and critically appraise the article and summarize his or her findings is acceptable. EBTP groups can be structured like journal clubs. The group should meet at a convenient time and location. A group facilitator who is enthusiastic, motivated, and knowledgeable about research and teaching issues should guide the group review of the selected research articles. Given the demanding schedules and workloads of nursing faculty, using technology such as videoconferencing would enable interested faculty to participate from distant locations. Having this forum to discuss educational research with others begins the conversation about use in teaching practice.

Providing support for those engaged in EBTP translation activities is critical. To truly embrace EBTP, resources need to be dedicated to support initiatives such as faculty development activities, workload release, reporting of EBTP in faculty meetings, and the collection of outcomes data. The review of EBTP research should not be a haphazard or isolated activity. To sustain a supportive culture, these efforts and resources need to be ongoing and become part of the values and norms at the institution.

INTEGRATING RESEARCH EVIDENCE INTO TEACHING PRACTICES

Nursing faculty will want to use the best available evidence to guide teaching practices; however, many nursing education studies have limitations such as single-site data collection, inadequate sample size, descriptive study designs lacking methodological rigor, and inadequate reporting of validated measures (Broome, Ironside, & McNelis, 2012; Mariani & Doolen, 2016; Yucha, Schneider, Smyer, Kowalski, & Stowers, 2011). These weaknesses may limit transferability and generalizability of the findings. Examining the results of a single study may not provide sufficient evidence to translate the findings into educational practices. The body of evidence in nursing education is developing. Some topics in nursing education research (e.g., simulation) have seen rapid growth. Although further research is needed to understand gaps in the simulation research, such as understanding the effectiveness of simulation on patient outcomes, the work in this area has expanded. When critically reviewing the simulation research, sufficient evidence existed to advance the NLN Jeffries Simulation framework to a mid-range theory that now facilitates best practices for teaching and learning to use simulation. However, not all areas in nursing education research have seen such rapid development.

There are some issues that faculty may want to consider as they look to the research to guide educational practices. Investigators can use rigorous research procedures that combine and compare the evidence from multiple studies. Using *comparative effectiveness research* (CER), which is "the systematic identification and synthesis of available research studies on a specific topic" (Katapodi & Northouse, 2011, p. 191) for comparative purposes, offers a more powerful approach, as it relies on all of the available evidence and not just the findings from a single study. It may also lead to better educational decision making and can ultimately impact educational practices. In the past, these CER techniques have not been widely used or supported sufficiently, yet they represent a reliable method of integrating evidence from multiple studies (Chalmers & Glasziou, 2009).

Before proceeding with a discussion of the steps of CER, it is important to understand some of the terminology associated with research synthesis and reporting. Table 8.3 presents the terms frequently associated with reviews of research literature, specifically literature review, integrative review, and systematic review. Most readers are probably familiar with the literature review that appears as part of a research report in journal articles. The traditional *literature review* describes and summarizes some of the literature that has been reported about a topic and presents a broad overview of the identified research. However, it does not represent a comprehensive collection of the publications about a topic nor does it represent a critical, systematic evaluation of the topic. It helps to identify important themes present in the nursing education literature, identify what has been studied, and illuminate existing gaps in knowledge (Polit & Beck, 2011).

TABLE 8.3

Research Evaluation Reviews in Nursing Education

Review Type	Description	Advantages	Disadvantage
Literature review	Descriptive summary of a limited group of references; usually narrow in scope or search	Provides background information or themes related to an educational topic	Lacks a priori standards for review Does not discuss magnitude of findings May not use a formalized, planned method for locating sources Process and outcomes may be imprecise
Integrative review	Summarizes diverse studies (descriptive and experimental) and theoretical articles	Synthesizes both empirical and theoretical literature related to educational topics Includes both experimental and nonexperimental studies	Poorly defined methods of analysis that may lack rigor and lead to bias
Systematic review	Critical review of studies with a specific study design May include a meta-analysis (findings of quantitative studies) or metasynthesis (findings from qualitative studies)	Uses precise search protocol and research techniques to comprehensively locate, examine, and synthesize existing educational research Findings considered robust and reliable	Limited experimental studies available in nursing education

(From Cooper, H. (2010). *Research synthesis and meta-analysis: A step-by-step approach*. Thousand Oaks, CA: Sage; Littell, J. H., Corcoran, J., & Pillai, V. (2008). *Systematic reviews and meta-analysis*. New York: Oxford University Press; and Polit, D. E., & Beck, C. T. (2011). *Nursing research: Generating and assessing evidence for nursing practice*. Philadelphia: Wolters Kluwer.)

Another term used when examining nursing education evidence is an *integrative review*. Typically, integrative reviews may include both theoretical and empirical literature, as well as research reports that use different data collection methods. Both experimental and nonexperimental research may be part of an integrative review. This broad inclusion of diverse literature can help to present an accurate state of the science of a nursing education topic. It can influence EBTP, help to develop theory, and may impact educational policy and practices, yet it also presents some challenges. Methods used to draw conclusions from this literature are not well defined and may lead to error (Cope, 2014; Whittemore & Knafl, 2005). Conversely, a systematic review follows a prescriptive format for the identification, review, and synthesis of the research. This method uses a protocol and employs a scientific design for identifying the relevant studies, examining them, and interpreting the data using a prescriptive protocol (Katapodi & Northouse, 2011). When using this approach, the findings are robust and

> **BOX 8.2**
>
> ## Research Synthesis Steps
>
> Formulate the problem.
> Search the literature.
> Gather information from studies.
> Evaluate the quality of the studies.
> Analyze and integrate the outcomes of the studies.
> Interpret the evidence.
> Present the results.
>
> _____
>
> *Source:* Cooper, H. (2010). *Research synthesis and meta-analysis: A step-by-step approach.* Thousand Oaks, CA: Sage.

reliable, and they offer a reproducible method of estimating the effect of an intervention (Aromataris & Pearson, 2014; Cope, 2014).

Nursing faculty wishing to use evidence to guide teaching practices may want to conduct a *systematic review* of evidence or read articles that provide a research synthesis systematic review. They will want to ensure that the review follows a specific and rigorous method. The steps for completing research synthesis are found in Box 8.2. Using these steps will help nursing faculty to evaluate the available evidence and aid decision making when considering the use of evidence in practice. Steps of the systematic review will be discussed in the following section.

Systematic Review Steps

The first step that nursing faculty will use when conducting a systematic review of educational research involves identifying the problem and formulating the research question. The question should clearly identify the topic of interest, population, and outcome (Higgins & Green, 2011). For example, Lee and Oh (2015) published a review that evaluated the effects of high-fidelity human simulation on cognitive, affective, and psychomotor outcomes of student learning using a CER technique. They identified the topic of interest (simulation), the population (nursing students), and outcomes (cognitive, affective, and psychomotor learning). Similarly, a systematic review by McCutcheon, Lohan, Traynor, and Martin (2015) evaluated the impact of online or blended learning versus face-to-face learning of clinical skills in undergraduate nurse education. This review clearly identifies the topic, population, and outcome under review and will be helpful for nursing faculty wishing to consider changes in education practice based on research.

Before proceeding with the next step in the review process, key inclusion and exclusion criteria or eligibility criteria for review must be established. Reviewers need to consider key search terms, dates for the reviews, and the types of studies that will be reviewed. Evidence hierarchies that rank evidence sources, such as those hierarchies published in research texts, are frequently used to identify or grade levels of evidence and can guide the type of evidence reviewed. Randomized control trials or single nonrandomized trials, usually considered a higher level of evidence than descriptive, correctional, or observational studies, are preferable when identifying best evidence (Polit & Beck, 2011). Another consideration the reviewer needs to make involves the type of publication. Nursing faculty conducting these reviews will need to determine if only peer-reviewed articles during a specified time period will be used or if other types of documents (e.g., dissertations, books, or conference proceedings) will be used in the analysis. Once these decisions have been made, the investigator should then perform a comprehensive literature search. Using key search words and Boolean operators in multiple databases will help to produce a comprehensive and extensive search. Reviewing article reference lists of the obtained studies will also provide a supplement to the electronic search and aid in identification of other key references. It is critical to ensure transparency and reproducibility of these search steps so that readers are clear about the techniques used. Once potential sources are identified, copies of the research reports are obtained, read, reviewed, and evaluated for quality. Standardized checklists, methods, or scoring systems are frequently used to appraise the study's quality (Porritt, Gomersall, & Lockwood, 2014; Risenberg & Justice, 2014). Usually, a team of investigators will scrutinize the research reports, extract and code information from the report, and document these key review items in a systematic and consistent way.

As part of the data review and extraction process, the investigator conducting a systematic review of quantitative education research would extract data from the identified reports, such as the methods used, the validity and reliability of the tools, and outcomes of the study. Statistical techniques may be employed to examine the pooled data from the quantitative research studies as part of a meta-analysis. A meta-analysis combines results from individual studies and estimates the overall effect size or "the strength and direction of the relationship between variables" (Munn, Tufanaru, & Aromataris, 2014, p. 50). As part of the systematic review, the use of statistical techniques can increase statistical power and offer more precise estimates of relationships between variables. This approach helps to synthesize the findings and examine the variables and effects of the interventions.

Similarly, single qualitative studies do not provide sufficient evidence to draw conclusions about teaching practices and their usefulness in educational practices. A metasynthesis is a systematic review with qualitative research. It enables comparison of findings from multiple qualitative studies (Sandelowski, Docherty, & Emden, 1997). Just like with meta-analysis, when using a metasynthesis approach, the investigator extracts the data using an appraisal method but with the aim of "enlarging the interpretive possibilities of findings and constructing larger narratives or general theories" (Sandelowski et al., 1997, p. 369). Paterson, Thorne, Canam, and Jillings (2001) suggest that there are three parts of the qualitative study analysis—metadata analysis, metamethod, and metatheory—that must occur before metasynthesis. They involve analysis of the qualitative research findings (metadata analysis), analysis of the qualitative research methods (metamethod), and analysis of theoretical and analytical frameworks of the qualitative research study (metatheory). This approach integrates qualitative findings, research methods, and frameworks from multiple studies; synthesizes the information; and arrives at a new interpretation of the pooled data (Munn et al., 2014; Polit & Beck, 2011). Many times when there is a sufficient body of qualitative research, the metastudy can lead to the development of a mid-range theory that may advance nursing science and nursing education.

Various methods can be used for these systematic reviews. Readers interested in conducting these comparative evaluation studies should consult references that can provide a more comprehensive explanation of these approaches. Investigators may want to consider using the Preferred Reporting Items for Systematic Reviews and Meta-Analyses (PRISMA) guidelines to enhance the quality and consistency of reporting and lessen reporting bias (Mohler, Liberati, Tetzlaff, & Altman, 2009). The PRISMA guidelines are available at www.prisma-statement.org. A review checklist, available on the PRISMA website, provides a standard format for review of the title, abstract, introduction, methods, results, discussion, and funding. Ultimately, the result of the review provides a synthesis of the studies and can lead to generalization of the pooled findings. Investigators can share the findings of the systematic review, thus helping faculty to support their practices.

Evidence for Educational Policy

Systematic reviews provide the best evidence for policy and program development because the findings from these reviews integrate evidence from multiple synthesized studies rather than relying on evidence from single studies (Nannini & Houde, 2010). Data from these systematic reviews may guide educational policies that direct action and allow for informed decision making. Relying on research evidence for policy creation is far superior to previously used methods, such as reliance on tradition or personal opinions. Evidence from nursing education studies can lead to the creation of policies at various levels. Policies can emerge at the local level, such as within a course or program of study. For example, academic policies and practices to deter cheating in nursing education were developed after a systematic review on the topic was completed (Stonecypher & Wilson, 2014). Policies based on research can also be created to address other teaching-learning challenges. Systematic reviews can direct other nursing program policies, such as those needed for course examinations, clinical performance, or student evaluations.

Rigorously conducted studies and comprehensive reviews of educational research topics can impact policy development at a broader level. Topics such as NCLEX® success or simulation use in nursing education lend themselves to review and policy development beyond an individual school. Nursing leaders can use the evidence from systematic reviews to inform educational practices at a national level. Research findings can help to direct state and national legislation and guidelines, such as regulations surrounding nursing clinical education and faculty.

The systematic review of simulation research offers an excellent example of how research can be used to advance nursing education, guide teaching practices, and impact theoretical thinking. The review of simulation literature led to the identification of themes, gaps in knowledge, and key issues. The NLN Jeffries Simulation framework also emerged from this work as a mid-range theory (Jeffries, 2016). Additionally, the NLN (2015) statement *A Vision for Teaching With Simulation* provides further guidance, identifies key strategies and resources, and offers a call to action for nurse leaders, faculty, and the NLN to further advance simulation. It would be expected that this work will impact policies in nursing programs.

Regardless of the level of policymaking, policy changes can be complex, as they can encompass attitudes, norms, and educational cultures. Usually, policy changes involve many stakeholders with vested interests. Since it can be a challenge to recommend and implement policy changes in nursing education, faculty need a sound rationale for the change, and research findings can provide that rationale. Research helps to focus on program improvement, enhance student quality, ensure that standards are met, and enhance evaluation processes.

CONCLUSIONS AND IMPLICATIONS

Evidence-based teaching is crucial for preparation of nursing students. However, for nurse faculty to be able to use evidence to guide their work, investigators must share their research. Publishing and presenting nursing education research findings will help to advance the science of nursing education, illuminate gaps in knowledge, and provide a launching point for future studies. Faculty need access to this critical research that will help to guide their work. The use of research in decision making about teaching and learning practices, curriculum development, program assessment, and evaluation will help to ensure quality in nursing education and ensure effective preparation of graduates ready for future practice.

References

Aromataris, E., & Pearson, A. (2014). The systematic review: An overview. *American Journal of Nursing, 114*(3), 53–58. doi:10.1097/01.NAJ.0000444496.24228.2c

Benner, P. (2013). Educating nurses: A call for radical transformation—how far have we come? *Journal of Nursing Education, 51*, 183–184. doi:10.3928/01484834-20120820-10

Benner, P., Sutphen, M., Leonard, V., & Day, L. (2009). *Educating nurses: A call for radical transformation.* San Francisco: Jossey-Bass.

Broome, M. E., Ironside, P. M., & McNelis, A. M. (2012). Research in nursing education: State of the science. *Journal of Nursing Education, 51*, 521–524. doi:10.3928/0148434-20120820-10

Chalmers, I., & Glasziou, P. (2009). Avoidable waste in the production and reporting of research evidence. *Lancet, 374*, 86–89. doi:10.1016/S0140-6736(09)60329-9

Cope, D. G. (2014). Analysis and use of different research review approaches in nursing. *Oncology Nursing Forum, 41*, 207–208. doi:10.1188/14.ONF.207-208

Dang, D., & White, K. (2012). Creating a supportive-evidence based environment. In S. Dearholt & D. Dang (Eds.), *Johns Hopkins nursing evidence-based practice models and guidelines* (pp. 163–193). Indianapolis, IN: Sigma Theta Tau International.

Gale, B. V. P., & Schaffer, M. A. (2009). Organizational readiness for evidence-based practice. *Journal of Nursing Administration, 39*, 91–97. doi:10.1097/NNA.0b013e318195a48d

Ginsberg, S. M., & Bernstein, J. L. (2011). Growing the scholarship of teaching and learning through institutional culture change. *Journal of the Scholarship of Teaching and Learning, 11*(1), 1–12.

Glasziou, P., Alman, D. G., Bossuyt, P., Boutron, I. L., Clarke, M., Julious, S., et al. (2014). Reducing waste from incomplete or unusable reports of biomedical research. *Lancet, 383*, 267–276. doi:10.1016/S0140-6736(13)62228.x

Hauck, S., Wisett, R. P., & Kuric, J. (2012). Leadership facilitation strategies to establish evidence-based practice in an acute care hospital. *Journal of Advanced Nursing, 69*, 664–674. doi:10.1111/j.1365-2648.2012.06053x

Higgins, J. P. T., & Green, S. (2011). *Cochrane handbook for systematic reviews of interventions.* Retrieved June 10, 2016, from http://handbook.cochrane.org

International Committee of Medical Journal Editors. (2011). *Uniform requirements for manuscripts submitted to biomedical journals: Writing and editing for biomedical publications.* Retrieved from http://www.icmje.org

Jeffries, P. R. (2016). *The NLN Jeffries Simulation theory.* Philadelphia: Wolters Kluwer.

Kalb, K. A., O'Conner-Von, S. K., Brockway, C., Rierson, C. L., & Sendelbach, S. (2015). Evidence-based teaching practice in nursing education: Faculty perspectives and practice. *Nursing Education Perspectives, 36,* 212–219. doi:10.5480/14-1472

Katapodi, M. C., & Northouse, L. L. (2011). Comparative effectiveness research: Using systematic reviews and meta-analyses to synthesize empirical evidence. *Research and Theory for Nursing Practice: An International Journal, 25,* 191–209. doi:10.1891/1541-6577.25.3.191

Lachance, C. (2014). Nursing journal clubs: A literature review on the effective teaching strategy for continuing education and evidence-based practice. *Journal of Continuing Education in Nursing, 45,* 559–565. doi:10.3928/00220124-20141120-01

Lang, T. A., & Altman, D. G. (2014). Basic statistical reporting for articles published in biomedical journals: The statistical analyses and methods in published literature or the SAMPL guidelines. *International Journal of Nursing Studies, 52,* 5–9. doi: 10.1016/j.ijnurstu.2014.009.006

Lee, J., & Oh, P. (2015). Effects of the use of high-fidelity human simulation in nursing education: A meta-analysis. *Journal of Nursing Education, 54,* 501–507. doi:10.3928/01484834-20150814-04

Mariani, B., & Doolen, J. (2016). Nursing simulation research: What are the perceived gaps? *Clinical Simulation in Nursing, 12,* 30–36. doi:10.1016/j.ecns.2015.11.004

McCutcheon, K., Lohan, M., Traynor, M., & Martin, D. (2015). A systematic review evaluating the impact of online or blended learning vs. face-to-face learning of clinical skills in undergraduate nurse education. *Journal of Advanced Nursing, 71,* 255–270. doi:10.1111/jan.12509

Melnyk, B. M., Fineout-Overholt, E., Gallagher-Ford, L., & Kaplan, L. (2012). The state of evidence-based practice in US nurses: Critical implications for nurse leaders and educators. *Journal of Nursing Administration, 42,* 410–417. doi:10.1097/NNA.0b013e3182664e0a

Mertler, C. A., & Charles, C. M. (2015). *Introduction to educational research.* Boston: Pearson Allyn & Bacon.

Mohler, D., Liberati, A., Tetzlaff, J., & Altman, D. G. (2009). Preferred reporting items for systematic reviews and meta-analyses: The PRISMA statement. *British Medical Journal, 339,* 332–336. doi:10.1136/bmj.b.2535

Munn, Z., Tufanaru, C., & Aromataris, E. (2014). Data extraction and synthesis. *American Journal of Nursing, 114*(7), 49–54. doi:10.1097/01.NAJ.0000451683.66447.89

Nannini, A., & Houde, S. C. (2010) Translating evidence from systematic reviews for policy makers. *Journal of Gerontological Nursing, 36*(6), 22–26. doi:10.3928/00989134-20100504-02

National League for Nursing. (2012). *NLN Vision: Transforming research in nursing education: A living document from the National League for Nursing.* Retrieved June 10, 2016, from http://www.nln.org/docs/default-source/about/nln-vision-series-%28position-statements%29/nlnvision_5.pdf?sfvrsn=4

National League for Nursing. (2015). *A vision for teaching with simulation.* NLN Vision Series. Retrieved June 10, 2016, from http://www.nln.org/docs/default-source/professional-development-programs/simulation-vision-statement3064b65c-78366c709642ff00005f0421.pdf?sfvrsn=2

Northam, S., Greer, D. B., Rath, L. O., & Toone, A. (2014). Nursing journal editor survey results to help nurses publish. *Nurse Educator, 39,* 290–297. doi:10.1097/NNE.0000000000000086

Nursing and Allied Health Resources Section Research Committee Journal Project Team.

(2012). *NAHRS 2012 selected list of nursing journals*. Retrieved June 10, 2016, from http://nahrs.mlanet.org/home/images/activity/nahrs2012selectedlistnursing.pdf

Oermann, M. H., & Hays, J. C. (2015). *Writing for publication in nursing*. New York: Springer.

Paterson, B. L., Thorne, S. E., Canam, C., & Jillings, C. (2001). *Meta-study of qualitative health research: A practice guide to meta-analysis and meta-synthesis*. Thousand Oaks, CA: Sage.

Patterson, B. J., & Klein, J. M. (2012). Evidence for teaching: What are faculty using? *Nursing Education Perspectives, 33*, 240–245. doi:10.5480/1536.5026-33.4.240

Polit, D. E., & Beck, C. T. (2011). *Nursing research: Generating and assessing evidence for nursing practice*. Philadelphia: Wolters Kluwer.

Porritt, K., Gomersall, J., & Lockwood, C. (2014). Study selection and critical appraisal: The steps following the literature search in a systematic review. *American Journal of Nursing, 114*(6), 47–52. doi:10.1097101.NAJ.0000450430.97383.64

Risenberg, L. A., & Justice, E. M. (2014). Conducting a successful systematic review of the literature, part 2. *Nursing, 44*(6), 23–26. doi:10.1097/01.NURSE.0000446641.02995.6a

Sandelowski, M., Docherty, S., & Emden, C. (1997). Qualitative metasynthesis: Issues and techniques. *Research in Nursing and Health, 20*, 365–371.

Stonecypher, K., & Wilson, P. (2014). Academic policies and practices to deter cheating in nursing education. *Nursing Education Perspectives, 35*, 167–179. doi:10.5480/12-1028.1

Whittemore, R., & Knafl, K. (2005). The integrative review: Updated methodology. *Journal of Advanced Nursing, 52*, 546–553. doi:10.1111/j.1365-2648.2005.03621.x

Yucha, C. B., Schneider, B. S. P., Smyer, T., Kowalski, S., & Stowers, E. (2011). Methodological quality and scientific impact of quantitative nursing education research over 18 months. *Nursing Education Perspectives, 32*, 362–368. doi:10.5480/1536-5026-32.6.362

9

Generating Simulation Evidence

Bette Mariani, PhD, RN

When writing this chapter, I reached out to a few well-respected simulation researchers and asked if they had something they would like to share with readers about the importance of simulation research to nursing education. I am pleased to include their insights throughout this chapter.

> *I cannot recall another point in the history of nursing education research in which formalized, concerted efforts to establish an evidence base for best practices to advance the science of nursing education has occurred as we are experiencing now with the output of evidence being generated through simulation-based research.* Mary Ann Cantrell, PhD, RN, FAAN (personal communication, December 17, 2015)

THE SCIENCE OF SIMULATION

Simulation is widely used as an educational strategy to teach undergraduate and graduate nursing students; it is an effective teaching and learning method when best practice guidelines are observed (Cant & Cooper, 2010). Although the science of simulation continues to evolve, nurse faculty need to have evidence that supports the educational outcomes of simulation as a teaching and learning strategy; ultimately, the goal is for the evidence to translate into the delivery of high-quality, safe patient care.

The purpose of this chapter is to provide an approach to a more rigorous methodology for simulation research that contributes to the science of nursing education. Currently, there is a plethora of single-site studies and research focused on student and faculty satisfaction with simulation (Mariani & Doolen, 2016), but as the science of nursing education in the area of simulation continues to advance, investigators must move beyond satisfaction and single-site studies to conduct research using a more rigorous design and measurable outcomes linking simulation as an educational strategy to student outcomes and potential to patient outcomes. Crawford and Lopez (2014) stated:

> research cannot be just a series of isolated activities, or tasks, such as surveys, interviews and observations; data collection and statistical analysis; improvement processes; or evidence-based practice (EBP) changes. Research is a rigorous, reproducible, and systematic process that may involve all or part of the above. (p. 1)

Recently, the landmark National Council of State Boards of Nursing (NCSBN) National Simulation Study (Hayden, Smiley, Alexander, Kardong-Edgren, & Jeffries, 2014) measured NCLEX® success based on the amount of time that nursing students spent in simulation. This study was important, as it was one of the first of its kind to demonstrate that the amount of time that students spent in simulation (10 percent, 25 percent, or 50 percent) did not have a statistically significant difference in their NCLEX results (Hayden, Smiley, et al., 2014). This finding supports the claim that simulation can be as effective as other methods of clinical education.

Simulation provides the opportunity for students to experience a representation of a real event within a safe learning environment (Gaba, 2004). In the past 10 to 15 years, simulation as a pedagogy to teach nursing students has grown exponentially. In 2010, Hayden reported that 87 percent of all nursing programs used some type of simulation (Hayden, 2010). As simulation requires a substantial investment in time, money, and resources, there is a growing demand for a return on that investment in many simulation centers; however, one of the challenges is guaranteeing quality and rigor in the delivery of simulation (Larsen & Schultz, 2014). When using simulation, whether for the purpose of formative assessment or summative evaluation, nurse faculty must take into consideration many of the same factors considered when conducting any type of research, such as who is the population of learners; what is/are the aim(s) or purpose(s) of the simulation; what is the setting; how will the outcomes be measured, including the validity and reliability of those measures; what is the intervention; what are the outcomes or results (Gaba, 2004; Shelestak & Voshall, 2014); and finally, how can those outcomes be used to advance simulation and inform the future of nursing education.

In many cases, simulation is a formative assessment for the students and serves the purpose of supplementing clinical and classroom learning experiences. However, the use of simulation for high-stakes testing is evolving (Rutherford-Hemming, Kardong-Edgren, Gore, Ravert, & Rizzolo, 2014), and as this develops, nurse faculty must be attentive to the delivery of simulation, the use of the evidence-based Standards of Best Practice (SOBPs) for simulation (International Nursing Association for Clinical Simulation and Learning, 2011, 2013; Decker et al., 2015; Lioce et al., 2015), and the types of evidence that are being used to validate simulation as an effective method to measure student performance. The International Nursing Association for Clinical Simulation and Learning (INACSL) SOBPs for simulation are an excellent resource for simulation specialists, nurse faculty, and investigators, providing guidelines for the consistency and quality of simulation, evaluation of outcomes, and continuous improvement of simulation programs (Rutherford-Hemming, Lioce, & Durham, 2015). These standards provide consistency in the delivery of simulation and prevent the variations in structure and process, which frequently influence student and program outcomes (Larsen & Schultz, 2014).

Simulation has been held to a high level of scrutiny, and has held up well. The unintended consequence of this scrutiny has been that traditional clinical education is now also being looked at rigorously, and is often found wanting. Suzie Kardong-Edgren, Phd, RN, FAAN, ANEF (personal communication, December 12, 2015)

RESEARCH PRIORITIES

Research priorities in simulation are available to guide nursing education research. Organizations such as the National League for Nursing (NLN), the INACSL, and the Society for Simulation in Healthcare (SSH) publish an ongoing and current list of research priorities on their websites that may guide investigators. Currently, research priorities are focused on multisite studies; studies using pilot-tested and valid scenarios, as well as reliable and valid instruments; studies that measure more significant and meaningful educational outcomes (beyond satisfaction, self-efficacy, and self-confidence); and research that can translate to patient outcomes. In reviewing these priorities, it is apparent that there is a need for more collaboration. Multisite studies require coordination and collaboration among investigators, nurse faculty, participants, and nursing education administration. Because of this need for a team approach, throughout this chapter, the term *investigator* is used to represent either an individual or team of investigators. The investigators conducting the study need the support of the administrators where the study will be conducted, the faculty teaching the students, the simulation specialists running the laboratory setting, and the students who will be participating in the simulations and the study. This collaboration of all stakeholders can move a rigorous simulation research agenda forward and hopefully provide a valuable contribution to the science of nursing education.

> *The use of simulation in nursing education is still being developed, making this not only an opportune time to conduct simulation research, but also a crucial time for rigorous research studies that establish evidence-based practices related to simulation.* Tonya Rutherford-Hemming, EdD, RN, ANP-BC, CHSE (personal communication, December 16, 2015)

FOUNDATION FOR CONDUCTING A SIMULATION STUDY

The various aspects of the research study design are crucial (some of which will be discussed later in the chapter), yet the foundation for a well-executed simulation study hinges on three notions: adherence to the INACSL SOBPs (2011, 2013; Decker et al., 2015; Lioce et al., 2015), a rigorous study design, and a project or strategic plan. Simulations have been widely used in nursing education for decades; however, when studying the outcomes of these educational interventions, it is crucial to employ stringent guidelines for their development, implementation, evaluation, and dissemination.

The INACSL SOBPs (2011, 2013; Decker et al., 2015; Lioce et al., 2015) were established for the purpose of providing best practices in simulation when designing, implementing, and evaluating simulation (Sittner et al., 2015); all are crucial when conducting a study to evaluate the outcomes of simulation. It is especially important to maintain best practices as investigators embark on the dialogue of utilizing simulation for high-stakes testing (Willhaus, Burleson, Palaganas, & Jeffries, 2014). Evidence supporting high-stakes testing must be obtained through rigorous, well-developed studies if outcomes related to student learning are to be determined from them. Adherence to the INACSL SOBPs is critical when conducting all simulations, as well as research including simulation. These standards provide the basis for well-developed simulations and include rationales, outcomes, criteria, and guidelines for various aspects of simulation, including but not limited to the participants, objectives, simulation design, facilitators, debriefing, interprofessional education, and assessment and evaluation. Of additional importance in conducting all simulations is the validation of simulation scenarios before they are used for measurement and evaluation in a study or for student evaluation (Shelestak & Voshall, 2014).

Next, a rigorous study design is imperative and includes three overarching components: development, implementation, and dissemination of results (Polit & Beck, 2012). Within these three components, seven clearly defined stages are delineated: conceptualization; design and planning; implementation of the study; collection, analysis, identification, and interpretation of the data; and dissemination of findings (Polit & Beck, 2012). Identifying a compelling problem is the catalyst for the study. A thorough review of the literature, background, and significance of the problem is required to validate the need for the study, as well as the relevance and generalizability of the results to a larger population. Next, the investigator has to select a theory or model to frame the study (further discussed in the next section). The simulation intervention should be well designed and based on the SOBPs, with clear identification of the comparison group, specification of the intervention being measured against, and how that will be identified. Then, the investigator must be clear about the outcome of interest and how it will be measured using valid and reliable instruments. This systematic inquiry in simulation, along with a rigorous study design, guides the investigator in creating new evidence or validating existing knowledge to advance the science of simulation and its application to nursing education. The final step of the research process is analyzing the results and disseminating the new knowledge (Polit & Beck, 2012).

Finally, as with any good project, a strategic plan is a critical step to ensure the success of the project (Kouzes & Pozner, 2012). In developing a plan, the investigator should identify key stakeholders and team members; the vision, goals, and objectives of the project; resources in terms of people, supplies, and funding; anticipated obstacles; how to engage the participants; and the evaluation or feedback mechanism. Frequently, this step of developing a strategic plan is overlooked; however, this plan is just as important to project success as developing the research question. A well-developed plan will assist the investigator in conducting a rigorous research project focused on the problem, and this plan can provide a blueprint for keeping the project on track, as well as provide valuable feedback to key stakeholders and team members, especially if funding has been obtained to conduct the research.

The process of conducting a simulation study is similar to conducting any other study in that there are elements imperative to a well-designed study. The goal of a simulation study is to create and disseminate evidence that contributes to the body of knowledge informing nursing education. There is overwhelming evidence supporting the use of simulation as a strategy for improving student outcomes (Adamson & Prion, 2016); however, simulation can be a costly investment in terms of time and resources. Therefore, it is imperative that, as a discipline, nurse faculty and investigators continue to contribute to the evidence supporting the use of simulation.

Creating the Evidence

At this point, the project plan is in place, the INACSL SOBPs are readily available, and the problem to be studied is well defined; at this point, the investigator is ready to

move forward in conducting a rigorous and well-design
this chapter is not meant to be a step-by-step guide on
various aspects of the research process are discussed, with
for a simulation study.

The Problem Statement

The problem statement should be well defined with literature to suppkground
and significance. Currently, a plethora of research exists on simulation, ɑ̣ɴough gaps in
the evidence remain (Lee & Oh, 2015; Yuan, Williams, Fang, & Ye, 2012; Mariani & Doolen, 2016), so
it is incumbent on investigators to thoroughly review the literature for gaps and conduct
a study that addresses these gaps rather than the areas that previously have been well
studied. A recent qualitative study (Mariani & Doolen, 2016) exploring the gaps and areas
of saturation in simulation research found that the areas of saturation were participant
and facilitator satisfaction, self-efficacy, and self-confidence, as well as descriptive and
single-site studies with a small number of participants. Furthermore, the gaps in simulation research included the need for more interventional studies with a rigorous design;
longitudinal, randomized controlled trials (RCTs) and large-scale studies; studies con-
firming reliability and validity of evaluation methods (Mariani & Doolen, 2016); and research
to provide support for linkages between simulation and improved patient outcomes
(Willhaus et al., 2014). The INACSL, NLN, and SSH identify research priorities; additionally,
investigators can use their own comprehensive review of the literature to inform their
research.

Theoretical or Conceptual Framework

Many simulation studies fall short in the area of the theoretical or conceptual framework
(Rourke, Schmidt, & Garga, 2010). From the start of designing a simulation study, it is critical
for investigators to include the theoretical framework as an integral part of the study.
The purpose of research is not only to answer a research question but also to build a
body of knowledge within a theoretical context to help investigators and simulation
users understand why or how the variables are related to each other and to help explain
or interpret results (Fain, 2015; Rourke et al., 2010). The theoretical or conceptual framework
is a key component and provides a structure or context for how the study is conducted
(Polit & Beck, 2012). Hayden, et al. (2014) cited theory-based simulation methods as crucial
to the success of simulation programs. Simulation studies should be conducted within
the context of a theoretical or contextual framework; some examples are learning,
instructional, technological, or self-efficacy theories (Rourke et al., 2010); Benner's model
of novice to expert practice (Benner, 1984); or the NLN Jeffries Simulation framework
(2007, 2016).

    A recent review by Fey, Gloe, and Mariani (2015) of 69 published articles in *Clinical
Simulation in Nursing* revealed that only 55 percent of the published studies during a
2-year period from January 2013 to December 2014 referenced a theoretical framework.
As the science of simulation continues to advance through research, there should be
an emphasis on the importance of the theoretical or conceptual framework as part of a
study, because theory as well as study outcomes are used to develop new knowledge.

...owing are good examples of how theory and/or framework can be used to ...simulation research. Zulkosky (2010) published a study exploring the impact of ...mulation on knowledge acquisition, satisfaction, and self-confidence. A strength of this study was the inclusion of two guiding theoretical frameworks. The first was the Nursing Education Simulation framework (Jeffries & Rogers, 2007), which the investigator used to guide the simulation development, and the Reflective Simulation framework (Alinier, 2008), which was used to provide structure during the simulation and to assist in fostering a deeper learning experience. In another example, Franklin, Sideras, Gubrud-Howe, and Lee (2014) conducted a study comparing the efficacy of three simulation preparation methods on novice nurses' competence in a multiple-patient simulation. The theoretical foundation for this study was Bandura's social cognitive theory.

Research Questions and Hypotheses

As with any study, the simulation study will be guided by the research questions and/or hypotheses. These should be formulated based on a thorough review of the literature, the identified problem, and the variables to be studied. The questions and hypotheses will drive the study design, sampling, data collection, and analysis (Fain, 2015). The research questions and hypotheses include the subjects to be studied (students, faculty, patients), the independent variable (the simulation intervention), and the dependent variables (the outcome being measured). The questions and hypotheses will drive the study design, and whether that is quantitative or qualitative in nature will be determined by the best method to answer the research question.

Methodology

The sample and setting, the simulation intervention (and how it will be validated), the type of measurement, and how the data will be collected and analyzed should be determined prior to conducting the study. Currently, there is a demand for more multisite studies in simulation. To this end, identifying the sample and setting of the study will require coordination and collaboration of effort among schools and colleges of nursing, which adds a level of complexity to the study.

A well-designed simulation study includes designing a simulation intervention according to the SOBPs for simulation design (Lioce et al., 2015). This includes a thorough assessment of the need for the simulation; measurable objectives; the format of the simulation; the actual clinical scenario or case; fidelity of the simulation; a guide for the facilitator; what will be included as briefing and debriefing; evaluation of the simulation; how the participants will be prepared; and finally, the testing (validity and reliability of the simulation). Although this appears to be a lengthy and unwieldy process, the rigor of the study depends on it. The investigator should take care to work through the various aspects of simulation design as an integral part of the research study and planning. Additionally, the investigator must have an understanding of when the simulation intervention will occur, how the investigator will control for other variables, who will facilitate it, how long the intervention will last, and how the facilitators will be trained.

Aronson, Glynn, and Squires (2013) conducted a quasiexperimental pretest-posttest pilot study to assess the preliminary effectiveness of a theory-based role-modeling intervention on enhancing student nurse competency in responding to a simulated response to rescue event. This pilot study is an example of an intervention study that met the crucial components of a simulation intervention study. The investigators provided a description of the need for the study; a theoretical framework; a thorough explanation of the intervention and dosing; description of the instruments, including reliability and validity; and application of this pilot study for future research. The thoroughness of this published study provides investigators the opportunity to replicate this study, and provides further evidence to support the role-modeling intervention. This detail and rigor contributes to opportunities for replication and collaboration and may form the foundation for conducting multisite studies—an area of simulation research that is sorely needed.

Multisite studies require various considerations (as well as a strategic plan), such as similarities or differences in academic programs, student populations, and simulation laboratories. Studies such as the one conducted by Aronson et al. (2013) open that door. Although multisite studies are important to advance the science of simulation, if these studies are conducted without attention to these critical aspects, it will be difficult to generalize and disseminate the results.

> *Using a standardized process for designing, implementing, debriefing, and evaluating simulation activities is key to having a successful and reliable simulation program. This process also supports successful simulation research activities.* Colleen Meakim, MSN, RN, CHSE (personal communication, December 18, 2015)

Measurement of the Outcomes

As simulation evolves, with an increasing focus on high-stakes testing, investigators must pay careful attention to factors such as simulation validity and fidelity, as well as instrument validity and reliability (Fey et al., 2015; Shelestak & Voshall, 2014). The fidelity of the simulation is particularly important, as the findings of studies using these simulations will inform the practice of nursing education where significant decisions about student performance may be made (Shelestak & Voshall, 2014). There is an emphasis on more RCTs and multisite studies; however, psychometric testing of simulations and instruments, single-site and pilot studies that are well designed for the purpose of providing validity and fidelity for simulation scenarios, and reliability and validity of instruments are needed. The findings and the dissemination of those findings from these pilot and single-site studies can be used for replication studies, as well as for larger multisite studies.

Although methods of assessing validity, such as content and construct validity, and reliability, including test-retest reliability and inter-rater reliability, are time intensive, evaluation of student performance in simulation is also complex and multidimensional (Adamson & Kardong-Edgren, 2012), making this a crucial step in advancing the science of simulation. These measures provide consistency in the delivery of the simulation intervention and measurement of outcomes, and they are important in producing valid and reliable results (Willhaus et al., 2014). It is not until validity and reliability are determined that the investigator should move forward with the intervention, data collection, and analysis of findings.

The Creighton Simulation Evaluation Instrument (C-SEI) (Todd, Manz, Hawkins, Parsons, & Hercinger, 2008) is an example of a research instrument with well-documented psychometric properties. It was developed to evaluate student participation in a simulated learning experience, and since then it has undergone rigorous psychometric testing and revision, with further reported psychometric analysis. The instrument was developed based on the core competencies of assessment, communication, critical thinking, and technical skills included in the *Essentials of Baccalaureate Education for Professional Nursing Practice* (American Association of Colleges of Nursing, 1998, 2008). The original instrument was pilot tested and had content validity testing by a panel of experts and an inter-rater reliability of 84.4 to 89.1 percent agreement overall for the entire instrument (Todd et al., 2008). Adamson, Gubrud-Howe, Sideras, and Lasater (2012) reported additional psychometrics on the C-SEI from multiple additional studies that used the instrument, which further confirmed its reliability (Adamson, 2011; Gubrud-Howe, 2008) with a Cronbach's alpha of .979 (Adamson et al., 2011).

Furthermore, a modified version of the C-SEI, the Creighton Competency Evaluation Instrument (C-CEI) was used for the NCSBN study (Hayden, Keegan, Kardong-Edgren, & Smiley, 2014) to evaluate competency in the simulation and clinical settings. Prior to using it in the NCSBN study, it was pilot tested across five schools of nursing to once again determine validity and reliability of the modified instrument. The content validity was considered acceptable, and the overall inter-rater reliability with the expert raters was 79.4 percent with a Cronbach's alpha of .90 (Hayden, Keegan, et al., 2014). Using instruments with good validity and reliability was crucial to maintaining the rigor of this landmark study and increasing confidence in the data to recommend policy change.

As interest in simulation for teaching and evaluation grows and the science matures, investigators are held to higher levels of evaluation to ensure that psychometric testing of instruments and validation and fidelity of simulations not only are addressed (Adamson, Kardong-Edgren, & Willhaus, 2013; Fey et al., 2015; Shelestak & Voshall, 2014) but also disseminated as investigators build a robust collection of evaluation instruments for simulation.

CHALLENGES OF CONDUCTING RESEARCH

Despite this need for research, and even the desire for nurse faculty and investigators to conduct studies to advance the science of simulation and inform nursing education, barriers exist. The most common challenges cited include funding; resources in terms of time, people, and space; a lack of research experience and mentors; a lack of standardization; and a lack of administrative support (Mariani & Doolen, 2016). Many of these challenges are very real for nurse faculty in the academic setting, especially with the competing responsibilities of teaching, scholarship, and service, as well as the shrinking number of faculty. The responsibility for advancing nursing education through research can be especially overwhelming for novice nurse faculty and investigators.

Another challenge is that simulation research relies heavily on the participation of student subjects, and many of these students are being asked to participate in multiple studies, so they may not be as willing to participate or as engaged as investigators would hope. This begs the questions of how much is enough and how to continue to advance the science without overburdening the students. As mentioned previously, the lack of standardization of curricula and simulations can present barriers to multisite studies; however, through more rigorous research and attention to the validity and fidelity of interventions, this barrier can be addressed.

Although it be may difficult for an individual investigator to address each of these challenges or barriers, with collaboration and attention to rigorously designed research, nurse faculty can create environments of scholarship that will help translate excellent nursing education into safe, quality patient care with excellent outcomes.

> *The use of simulation in nursing education is increasing without much consideration on how it will be appropriately integrated into curricula or how it will improve student learning outcomes. Simulation based learning activities and evaluation strategies need to be thoughtfully constructed and based on established guidelines, best practices and the growing evidence derived from rigorously designed research.* Barbara Aronson, PhD, RN, CNE (personal communication, February 10, 2016)

ADVANCING THE SCIENCE THROUGH EVIDENCE AND RESEARCH

As nursing education continues to move in the direction of increasing the amount of simulation in undergraduate education, it is imperative to elevate the level of rigor in the evidence that is used to support this practice. Studies and simulations that lack quality can hinder the use of simulation to advance the science of simulation and nursing education (Fey et al., 2015), and it is imperative that the fidelity, validity, and reliability of the simulations used as a teaching-learning strategy are addressed and receive just as much rigor as they do in the research process (Shelestak & Voshall, 2014). Not only is the use of simulation important, but the techniques employed in simulation and simulation research can improve the pedagogy of simulation for faculty and students (Starkweather & Kardong-Edgren, 2008) and contribute to best teaching practices. These best practices in simulation can contribute to consistency in the curriculum for all students, especially where they lack those opportunities in the clinical setting (Brewer, 2011), particularly in specialty areas.

The NLN identified the use of instructional technologies such as simulated learning as one of its priorities for research in nursing education (Gresley, 2009). This, as well as the priorities set forth by INACSL, emphasizes the importance of research to support educational outcomes of simulation, such as student learning and improvement in the educational process, and the transition to practice, such as patient outcomes or patient safety. Nurse faculty engaged in the scholarship of simulation research contribute to achieving excellence in nursing education and are making great strides in addressing some aspect of each of the eight NLN Nurse Educator Core Competencies (Halstead, 2009). These are supported by (a) facilitating learning through evidence-based teaching strategies such as simulation, using assessment and evaluation to make meaningful decisions about student learning in simulation; (b) contributing to curriculum design by participating in simulation development and testing, functioning as a change agent to bring evidence-based simulation to the curriculum, participating in continuous improvement while growing in the role of teaching, scholarship, and service, and engaging in scholarship to advance the science of simulation; and (c) functioning within the educational environment by being knowledgeable and sensitive to the trends and issues affecting nursing education, especially those related to the contribution of simulation to achieving excellence in nursing education.

Simulation as a pedagogical approach to educating nurses is here to stay. As nursing education moves into the next decade, there will be an increasing demand for evidence supporting simulation as a teaching-learning strategy with positive outcomes in terms of student outcomes, patient outcomes, and patient safety. As the discussion surrounding high-stakes testing and evaluation continues, it will be incumbent on nurse investigators and nurse faculty to conduct rigorous studies with attention to careful strategic planning, as well as the use of well-designed, tested, and facilitated simulations; careful implementation; attention to fidelity; and valid and reliable measurement and evaluation. These measures will provide the validity and reliability to be able to use simulation as a method for evaluating student performance (Rizzolo, Kardong-Edgren, Oermann, & Jeffries, 2015).

> Simulation-based education, like all educational methodologies, should be based on the best available evidence. Drawing on a rich body of evidence from diverse fields as well as research in healthcare simulation, the INACSL Standards of Best Practice: Simulation[SM], provide guidance to healthcare simulation educators in all disciplines. Mary Fey, PhD, RN, CHSE (personal communication, February 16, 2016)

CONCLUSIONS AND IMPLICATIONS

Simulation continues to be an effective teaching strategy for validation and evaluation of skills, and it provides a safe learning environment for the development of clinical judgment, decision making, and problem solving. Nurse faculty and investigators can be at the forefront in conducting rigorous, quality, theory-based simulation research. Dissemination of findings through national and international conferences and publications is imperative but all too often is a missing link to creating evidence and knowledge to advance the science of nursing education.

References

Adamson, K. A. (2011). *Assessing the reliability of simulation evaluation instruments used in nursing education: A test of concept study.* Doctoral dissertation. Available from ProQuest Dissertations and Theses database. UMI No. 3460357

Adamson, K. A., Gubrud-Howe, P., Sideras, S., & Lasater, K. (2012). Assessing the reliability, validity, and use of the Lasater clinical judgment rubric: Three approaches. *Journal of Nursing Education, 51*, 66–73. doi:10.3928/01484834-20111130-03

Adamson, K., & Kardong-Edgren, S. (2012). A method and resources for assessing the reliability of simulation evaluation instruments. *Nursing Education Perspectives, 33*, 334–339. doi:10.5480/1536-5026-33.5.334

Adamson, K. A., Kardong-Edgren, S., & Willhaus, J. (2013). An updated review of published simulation evaluation instruments. *Clinical Simulation in Nursing, 9*, e393–e400. doi:10.1016/j.ecns.2012.09.004

Adamson, K. A., Parsons, M. E., Hawkins, K., Manz, J. A., Todd, M., & Hercinger, M. (2011). Reliability and internal consistency findings from the C-SEI.

Journal of Nursing Education, 50, 583–586. doi:10.3928/01484834-20110715-02

Adamson, K., & Prion, S. (2016). Making sense of methods and measurement: Cost-effectiveness research, *Clinical Simulation in Nursing, 12*, 49–50. doi:10.1016/j.ecns.2015.10.009

Alinier, G. (2008). Learning through play: Simulation scenario = obstacle course + treasure hunt. In R. Kyle, & W. B. Murray (Eds.), *Clinical simulation: Operations, engineering and management* (pp. 745–749). Burlington, MA: Academic Press.

American Association of Colleges of Nursing (1998). *The essentials of baccalaureate education for professional nursing practice.* Washington, DC: Author.

American Association of Colleges of Nursing (2008). *The essentials of baccalaureate education for professional nursing practice.* Washington, DC: Author.

Aronson, B., Glynn, B., & Squires, T. (2013). Effectiveness of a role-modeling intervention on student nurse simulation competency. *Clinical Simulation in Nursing, 9*(4), e121–e126. doi:10.1016/j.ecns.2011.11.005

Benner, P. (1984). *From novice to expert: Excellence and power in clinical nursing practice.* Menlo Park, CA: Addison-Wesley.

Brewer, E. (2011). Successful techniques for using human patient simulation in nursing education. *Journal of Nursing Scholarship, 43*, 311–317. doi:10.1111/j.1547-5069.2011.01405.x

Cant, R., & Cooper, S. (2010). Simulation-based learning in nurse education: Systematic review. *Journal of Advanced Nursing, 66*, 3–15. doi:10.1111/j.1365-2648.2009.05240.x

Crawford, C., & Lopez, C. (2014). The research process and simulation in nursing. What it is and what it is not. *Journal for Nurses in Professional Development, 30*, 127–133. doi:10.1097/NND.0000000000000019

Decker S. I., Anderson M., Boese T., Epps C., McCarthy J., Motola I., et al. (2015). Standards of Best Practice: Simulation Standard VIII: Simulation-enhanced interprofessional education (sim-IPE).

Clinical Simulation in Nursing, 11, 293–297. doi:10.1016/j.ecns.2015.03.010

Fain, J. (2015). *Reading, understanding, and applying nursing research* (4th ed.). Philadelphia: F. A. Davis.

Fey, M. K., Gloe, D., & Mariani, B. (2015). Assessing the quality of simulation-based research articles: A rating rubric. *Clinical Simulation in Nursing, 11*, 496–504. doi:10.1016/j.ecns.2015.10.005

Franklin, A. E., Sideras, S., Gubrud-Howe, P., & Lee, C. S. (2014). Comparison of expert modeling versus voice-over PowerPoint lecture and presimulation readings on novice nurses' competence of providing care to multiple patients. *Journal of Nursing Education, 53*, 615–622. doi:10.3928/01484834-20141023-01

Gaba, D. (2004). The future vision of simulation in healthcare. *Quality and Safety in Healthcare, 13*(Suppl. 1), 2–10. doi:10.1136/qshc.2004.009878

Gresley, R. (2009). Building a science of nursing education. In C. Shultz (Ed.), *Building a science of nursing education: Foundation for evidence-based teaching-learning* (pp. 1–13). New York: National League for Nursing.

Gubrud-Howe, P. (2008). *Development of clinical judgment in nursing students: A learning framework to use in designing and implementing simulated learning experiences.* Unpublished doctoral dissertation. Portland State University, Portland, OR.

Halstead, J. (2009). Well-prepared faculty: Needed to achieve excellence in nursing education. In M. Adams & T. Valiga (Eds.), *Achieving excellence in nursing education* (pp. 29–42). New York: National League for Nursing.

Hayden, J. (2010). Use of simulation in nursing education: National survey results. *Journal of Nursing Regulation, 1*(3), 52–57. doi:10.1016/S2155-8256(15)30335-5

Hayden, J., Keegan, M., Kardong-Edgren, S., & Smiley, R. A. (2014). Reliability and validity testing of the Creighton competency evaluation instrument for use in the NCSBN National Simulation Study. *Nursing*

Education Perspectives, 35, 244–252. doi:10.5480/13-1130.1

Hayden, J. K., Smiley, R. A., Alexander, M. A., Kardong-Edgren, S., & Jeffries, P. R. (2014). The NCSBN National Simulation Study: A longitudinal, randomized, controlled study replacing clinical hours with simulation in prelicensure nursing education. *Journal of Nursing Regulation, 5*(2), S3–S40. doi:10.1016/S2155-8256(15)30062-4

International Nursing Association for Clinical Simulation and Learning. (2011). Standards of Best Practice: Simulation. *Clinical Simulation in Nursing, 7*(4), Si–S19. doi:10.1016/S1876-1399(11)00109-5

International Nursing Association for Clinical Simulation and Learning. (2013). Standards of Best Practice: Simulation. *Clinical Simulation in Nursing, 9*(6), Si–S32. doi:10.1016/j.ecns.2013.05.008

Jeffries, P. R. (Ed.). (2007). *Simulations in nursing education: From conceptualization to evaluation.* New York: National League for Nursing.

Jeffries, P. R. (2016). *The NLN Jeffries Simulation theory.* Philadelphia: Wolters Kluwer.

Jeffries, P., & Rogers, K. J. (2007). Theoretical framework for simulation design. In P. Jeffries (Ed.), *Simulation in nursing education* (pp. 21–33). New York: National League for Nursing.

Kouzes, J., & Posner, B. (2012). *The leadership challenge workbook* (3rd ed.). San Francisco: Jossey-Bass.

Larsen, T. A., & Schultz, M. A. (2014). Transforming simulation practices: A quest for return on expectations. *Clinical Simulation in Nursing, 10*, 626–629. doi:10.1016/j.ecns.2014.09.004

Lee, J., & Oh, P. (2015). Effects of the use of high-fidelity human simulation in nursing education: A meta-analysis. *Journal of Nursing Education, 54*, 501–507. doi:10.3928/01484834-20150814-04

Lioce, L., Meakim, C. H., Fey, M. K., Chmil, J. V., Mariani, B., & Alinier, G. (2015). Standards of Best Practice: Simulation Standard IX: Simulation design. *Clinical*

Simulation in Nursing, 11, 309–315. doi:10.1016/j.ecns.2015.03.005

Mariani, B., & Doolen, J. (2016). Nursing simulation research: What are the perceived gaps? *Clinical Simulation in Nursing, 12*(1), 30–36. doi:10.1016/j.ecns.2015.11.004

Polit, D., & Beck, C. (2012). *Nursing research: Generating and assessing evidence for nursing practice* (9th ed.). Philadelphia: Wolters Kluwer Health/Lippincott Williams & Wilkins.

Rizzolo, M. A., Kardong-Edgren, S., Oermann, M., & Jeffries, P. (2015). The National League for Nursing Project to explore the use of simulation for high-stakes assessment: Process, outcomes, and recommendations. *Nursing Education Perspectives, 36*, 299–303. doi:10.5480/15-1639

Rourke, L., Schmidt, M., & Garga, N. (2010). Theory-based research of high fidelity simulation use in nursing education: A review of the literature. *Journal of Nursing Education Scholarship, 7*(1), 1–14. doi:10.2202/1548-923X.1965

Rutherford-Hemming, T., Kardong-Edgren, S., Gore, T., Ravert, P., & Rizzolo, M. A. (2014). High-stakes evaluation: Five years later. *Clinical Simulation in Nursing, 10*, 605–610. doi:10.1016/j.ecns.2014.09.009

Rutherford-Hemming, T., Lioce, L., & Durham, C. (2015). Implementing the Standards of Best Practice for simulation. *Nurse Educator, 40*(2), 96–100. doi:10.1097/NNE.0000000000000115

Shelestak, D., & Voshall, B. (2014). Examining validity, fidelity, and reliability of human patient simulation. *Clinical Simulation in Nursing, 10*(5), e257–e260. doi:10.1016/j.ecns.2013.12.003

Sittner, B., Aebersold, M., Paige, J., Graham, L. Schram, A. Decker, S., et al. (2015). INACSL standards for best practice in simulation: Past, present, and future. *Nursing Education Perspectives, 35*, 294–298. doi:10.5480/15-1670

Starkweather, A. R., & Kardong-Edgren, S. (2008). Diffusion of innovation : Embedding simulation into nursing curricula. *International Journal of Nursing, 5*(1), 1–11. doi:10.2202/1548-923X.1567

Todd, M., Manz, J., Hawkins, K., Parsons, M., & Hercinger, M. (2008). The development of a quantitative evaluation tool for simulations in nursing education. *International Journal of Nursing Education Scholarship, 5*(1), 1–17. doi:10.2202/1548-923X.1705

Willhaus, J., Burleson, G., Palaganas, J., & Jeffries, P. (2014). Authoring simulations for high-stakes student evaluation. *Clinical Simulation in Nursing, 10,* e177–e182. doi:10.1016/j.ecns.2013.11.006

Yuan, H. B., Williams, B. A., Fang, J. B., & Ye, Q. H. (2012). A systematic review of selected evidence on improving knowledge and skills through high-fidelity simulation. *Nurse Education Today, 32,* 294–298. doi:10.1016/j.nedt.2011.07.010

Zulkosky, K. D. (2010). Simulation use in the classroom: Impact on knowledge acquisition, satisfaction, and self-confidence. *Clinical Simulation in Nursing, 8*(1), e25–e33. doi:10.1016/j.ecns.2010.06.003

10

Creating Evidence for Distance Education in Nursing

Barbara Manz Friesth, PhD, RN

Anne M. Krouse, PhD, MBA, RN-BC

Distance education (DE) has been a part of higher education for decades, with its initiation dating back to the late 1800s (Armstrong, Gessner, & Cooper, 2000). In the most general terms, DE is defined as education that occurs with a physical separation between the faculty member and the student. The technologies utilized in DE have changed dramatically over the years, matching the technology of the day and ranging from books, radio, telephone, mail, television, cable, satellite, all the way to computers and mobile devices. Around the mid-1990s, coinciding with the advent of the Internet and more widespread use of home computers, DE over the Internet began to see much more significant growth and traction. The growth in DE has continued at a rapid pace ever since, with the most recent analysis of data showing that one in seven students in higher education are attending exclusively at a distance (Poulin, 2015). Even more staggering are the numbers of learners who are taking at least one course from a distance, which totals in excess of 5.25 million learners in the United States alone (Allen & Seaman, 2015).

The purpose of this chapter is to examine opportunities for educational research in nursing related to learning at a distance and online instruction. Definitions and a common language for the terms *online* and *distance education* will be delineated. A review of current priorities for research, theoretical perspectives, and methodological approaches will also be presented. Challenges facing investigators researching the online or DE environment will be discussed, as well as new and emerging technologies that may impact researching of DE in the future.

This chapter will not address the equivalency of DE to traditional face-to-face courses or programs. Numerous studies comparing the equivalency of DE to traditional formats have been conducted, albeit largely in other disciplines, with the results demonstrating equivalent outcomes regardless of format (Bernard et al., 2004; Means, Toyama, Murphy, & Baki, 2013; Sitzmann, Kraiger, Stewart, & Wisher, 2006; U.S. Department of Education, 2009; Zhao, Lei, Yan, Lai, & Tan, 2005). In addition, accreditation standards require that nursing programs delivered completely or partially through DE must meet the same "support standards and accreditation criteria as programs provided in face-to-face formats" (American Association of Colleges of Nursing, 2007). Because of the overwhelming evidence of equivalency and the widespread acceptance of DE, this chapter will focus on research agendas and priorities that extend beyond the equivalency question.

A COMMON LANGUAGE FOR DISTANCE EDUCATION AND ONLINE LEARNING

Over the years, several terms have been used nearly synonymously to describe learning at a distance over the Internet, including *distance education, distance accessible, e-learning, online,* and *web based.* In more recent years, with widespread availability of high-speed Internet, synchronous video has begun to blur the lines of what is meant by online versus blended or hybrid learning. The confusion over DE and online definitions is exacerbated by lack of consistency across federal, state, and accrediting agencies definitions. In addition, many universities and colleges have adopted their own definitions for use in coding individual courses. To further complicate the discussion, the definitions for what constitutes DE, online, or some other format vary depending on whether the discussion is about individual courses or entire academic programs.

The federal government only provides a definition for DE, not for online education. The main criteria of the federal definition of DE includes the separation of the teacher from the student; substantive interaction between the faculty and student; and a list of inclusive technologies that may be used to facilitate the interaction, including the Internet. The Higher Learning Commission (HLC) is one of the accrediting agencies for degree-granting postsecondary educational institutions, specifically in the North Central region of the United States. The HLC definition of DE is identical to that of the federal government; however, the HLC further provides definitions for DE courses and programs. According to the HLC, DE courses involve instruction where the majority (75 percent or greater) is delivered at a distance. Their definition of distance programs, however, requires that at least 50 percent or greater of the courses are taken at a distance. As there are several regional and national accrediting agencies in the United States, there are numerous variations on the definition of DE across agencies.

In addition to the federal, national, and regional accrediting bodies' definitions, each state commission for higher education may also have separate definitions for what constitutes a course or program delivered at a distance. A simple web search for online or DE programs in nursing results in a wide variety of courses and programs delivered in a variety of modalities. There is little consistency in either the lay or research literature on definitions for DE or online education. Because of the variability in definitions and concern for the ability to share research findings across modalities, Mayadas, Miller, and Sener (2015) from the Online Learning Consortium (OLC) have proposed definitions for a common language when referring to DE. The proposed language includes definitions for both the course and program level, and are based on delivery modality, percentage of time in a given modality, and flexibility of the learners' schedule. The authors proposed seven categories for representation of course-level instruction and include the terms *classroom course, synchronous distributed course, web-enhanced course, blended* or *hybrid classroom course, blended* or *hybrid online course, online course,* and *flexible mode course.* Table 10.1 summarizes the definitions for each of the proposed course definitions, including the modality and percentage of time devoted to the modality, as well as the level of flexibility of the course offering.

TABLE 10.1

Summary of Course Level Definitions

Type of Course	Definition
Classroom	Traditional face-to-face classroom based course scheduled around class meetings.
Synchronous Distributed	Courses meet real time using web-based, synchronous technologies. May occur with a mix of on-campus and at a distance students.
Web-Enhanced	Some online Internet component required for an otherwise Classroom based course. The amount of required Internet based work should not exceed 20% of total class time.
Blended or Hybrid Classroom	Online or Internet based activities replaces a significant percent of required face-to-face classroom sessions.
Blended or Hybrid Online	Majority of course takes place online over the Internet, with very little required synchronous or face-to-face instruction.
Online	All instruction occurs via the Internet online, with no required synchronous or on-campus course requirements.
Flexible Mode	The course is offered in more than one delivery mode, offering students a choice in preferred modality.

The terms used for program-level definitions are similar to the course-level definitions and are broken into four categories based on the mix of traditional classroom courses versus other modalities (Mayadas et al., 2015). The proposed terms for program-level definitions include *classroom program, multiformat program, blended program,* and *online program.* Table 10.2 summarizes the definitions for each of the program-level definitions.

Given the concern for consistency in language related to DE and online education in nursing, it is essential that investigators in nursing education begin to use a common language for these modalities in research and when reporting results. The authors of this chapter encourage the use of the proposed definitions from Mayadas et al. (2015)

TABLE 10.2

Summary of Program Level Definitions

Type of Program	Definition
Classroom Program	The overall program may include a mix of types of courses, but all courses require some face-to-face classroom sessions.
Multi-Format Program	The program uses a mix of classroom courses with a variety of different delivery modes.
Blended Program	A significant portion of the credits are offered online, with up to 30% of the curriculum offered as face-to-face or blended courses.
Online Program	All required credit hours are offered via fully online courses.

and the OLC, as well as those summarized in this chapter. These definitions may morph over time with changes by regulatory agencies, state, and federal definitions, as well as impact by changes in evolving technology. At a minimum, for the ability to compare and contrast research results across modalities, and for inclusion purposes in meta-analyses, a clear definition of the modality of instruction is required.

NURSING EDUCATION RESEARCH PRIORITIES

The recommended priorities for research in nursing education related to DE have been gleaned from a variety of sources. The National League for Nursing (NLN) published priorities for research in nursing education, including increasing multisite and multimethod research designs, the use of meta-analysis and metasynthesis methodologies, and the examination of the use of technology on student learning (National League for Nursing, 2016). The NLN's latest agenda is consistent with prior calls to increase the rigor of research in nursing education (Broome, Ironside, & McNelis, 2012; Yucha, Schneider, Smyer, Kowalski, & Stowers, 2011), including the use of multisite studies, the use of randomized controlled trials, improved quality of evaluation instruments, increased sample sizes, and a focus on outcomes beyond satisfaction. The use of the aforementioned discussion of definitions regarding DE and online learning is especially pertinent given the call for more multisite studies. The consistency in language is essential to ensure the equivalency of the comparisons. In addition, given the ever-changing nature of technology in DE, the need to evaluate the effectiveness of new technologies and their effect on student learning will be ongoing.

DISTANCE EDUCATION RESEARCH

Research in distance learning poses several opportunities and challenges for investigators, not unlike other forms of educational research. The contextual variations associated with teacher and learner characteristics and the educational environment confounds even the most well-designed research studies. Research studies, particularly those examining differences between face-to-face and online delivery methods, pose challenges related to the rigor of the study, particularly when students may have inherently different characteristics based on their choice of course delivery format. Multisite studies pose additional challenges because of differences in the faculty, the learners themselves, and the online learning environment. The following sections will provide guidance on the use of a theoretical or conceptual framework, the design of the study, measurement, and future areas for research.

THEORETICAL OR CONCEPTUAL FRAMEWORKS

A criticism of DE studies in nursing education is the lack of theoretical frameworks driving research questions and design (Patterson & Krouse, 2012; Thurmond, 2002), as well as an analysis of how the findings from the resulting data analysis fit with the theoretical underpinnings. A variety of theories have been posed for their use in research in nursing education and DE, including constructivism, a systems model, a theoretical model of supportive learning, and Astin's Input-Environment-Output (I-E-O) conceptual model (Patterson & Krouse, 2012). A broader look at DE education outside of nursing reveals a broader array of theories utilized in other disciplines more extensively to guide DE research (Bozkurt et al., 2015), with the most commonly reported theories including community of inquiry, collaborative learning, constructivism, connectivism, transactional distance theory, activity theory, social presence theory, and self-regulated learning theory. Some of these theories have been reported in the nursing literature; however, the use of conceptual frameworks or theory in general remains an area that could be improved. The relevancy of these theories to nursing and the science of nursing education warrants additional consideration.

DESIGN

Good research starts with a well-developed research design that is appropriate for the research question. The most common designs used in DE research in nursing are descriptive, quasiexperimental, and qualitative. Meta-analyses and metasyntheses have also been used to provide a synthesis of prior research. The following sections discuss the use of the design in DE studies and provide examples of DE studies in nursing or education that have used those designs.

Descriptive Designs

Many studies in DE research have employed a *descriptive* design, particularly when examining student characteristics, faculty characteristics, student perceptions, student engagement, and outcomes such as student satisfaction. Although these data are important to understand the contexts in which distance learning is occurring, it is limited in its ability to provide evidence to support nursing education.

Correlational designs may also be used to examine the relationships between variables. There is no attempt to determine causality in correlational research (Grove, Burns, & Gray, 2012). For example, the relationship between computer proficiency and student persistence in online learning may be examined to attempt to understand why some students are more likely to continue in their DE program. Correlational designs may be used for description, prediction, or model testing.

Comparative descriptive designs may be employed to examine differences in certain variables using two or more groups. An example of this is the analysis of student engagement in DE between two groups of students who either are taking a class using a hybrid format or a completely online design (Gliner, Morgan, & Leech, 2009). *Causal comparative* designs attempt to explain a cause-and-effect relationship between variables. With this type of design, there are at least two groups without random assignment to those groups. For example, many studies over the past decade have compared outcomes among those students participating in DE and traditional classes. The students have generally self-selected the class section in which to enroll. Student outcomes are then measured and differences examined among the groups. The causal effect of the type of class, the independent variable (DE or traditional), is then examined in relation to the achievement of student learning outcomes.

One of the concerns of correlational, comparative descriptive, and causal comparative designs is that the observed relationship is spurious, meaning that because the independent variable is not manipulated, the results may be due to a third variable that was not studied (Johnson, 2000). Careful selection of the variables to be studied based on theory and/or a robust literature review will minimize the likelihood of this occurring. Additionally, in comparing results from different groups, particularly given that there will be self-selection into those groups, the investigator should carefully consider collecting data on characteristics on which the participants can be matched across groups or to describe the sample after the completion of the study, demonstrating equivalence after the fact.

Examples of Descriptive Studies

Cameron (2013) conducted a study using archival data to compare characteristics of graduate admission and graduating grade point averages (GPAs), and family nurse practitioner (FNP) certification first-time examination pass rates among students participating in an online and face-to-face master of science in nursing program. The face-to-face students had statistically significant higher bachelor of science in nursing (BSN) GPAs ($p = .003$) and higher admission scores ($p = .006$) than the online applicants. No differences were found in admitted student GPAs, GPAs at the completion of the program, and FNP certification rates.

Quasiexperimental Designs

Because true experimental designs require random assignment to groups, most educational research in DE in nursing examining the effect of an independent variable that can be manipulated on a dependent variable is *quasiexperimental.* Sampling plans in nursing education research a as whole tend to be convenience samples where random assignment is difficult to operationalize. The weakest of the quasiexperimental designs is the *one-group posttest-only* design. This is a limited design in that it becomes almost impossible to make the conclusion that the results of the posttest were due to the intervention (Gliner et al., 2009). This type of study has been used to examine student outcomes such as satisfaction or knowledge after participation in an online learning activity.

A *one-group pretest-posttest* design is slightly more rigorous with the inclusion of a pretest measurement. However, this design still lacks the inclusion of a control group; therefore, changes in posttest scores may not necessarily be due to the intervention. Rather, the effect of extraneous variables may have actually been the influence on posttest scores (Gliner et al., 2009). Shadish, Cook, and Campbell (2002) recommend the inclusion of additional dependent variables in the research design to increase the confidence that the change in the posttest scores was more likely to be a result of the intervention, as not all of the dependent variables would be expected to change. An example of the use of this type of design in DE would be an online learning intervention that was designed to change attitudes. Student attitudes would be measured prior to the online intervention and at completion.

The *posttest-only nonequivalent comparison group* design is often used when comparing outcomes among face-to-face and DE classes. The outcomes measured most often are subject matter knowledge and student satisfaction. Investigators use this type of design because random assignment is not a possibility (Gliner et al., 2009). The threat is that there are significant differences between the groups that may have a direct influence on the outcomes. Information about participant demographics should be collected to assess for group equivalence.

A *pretest-posttest nonequivalent* group design is stronger in that there is an intervention and a control group, and the dependent variables are measured and compared at both points in the study (Gliner et al., 2009). Careful consideration of demographic variables to be measured should occur so that group equivalence can be examined after data collection.

Example of a Quasiexperimental Study

Wells and Dellinger (2011) used a quasiexperimental posttest-only design to study the effect of the learning environment (Internet only, compressed video remote site, and compressed video host site) on final course grades, perceived learning, feelings of connectedness, learner-to-learner interaction, learner-to-instructor interaction, and learner-to-system interaction among 49 graduate nursing students. The Leaner-Interaction model was used to guide the study. The compressed video host site was the control group in this study. The interaction variables were measured using the Learner Interaction Tool, and the Classroom Community Scale (CSS) was used to measure feelings of connectedness. No significant differences were found for any of the dependent variables among the groups. A positive correlation was found between perceived learning and learner-instructor interaction ($r = .54$; $p < .000$) and between perceived learning and learner-system interaction ($r = .38$; $p = .01$).

Hunter and Krantz (2010) used a quasiexperimental pretest-posttest control group design to examine the influence of instructional delivery mode (online or face-to-face) on student cultural competence scores. The investigators used constructivist learning theory to guide the development of the course. Cultural competency was measured using the total and subscale score of the Inventory for Assessing the Process of Cultural Competence Among Healthcare Professionals–Revised (IAPCC-R). The findings revealed a significant increase in cultural competency scores ($p < .001$) for all students after completion of the course. The course delivery method was not found to have an influence on cultural competency scores.

Experimental Designs

A true *experimental design* is the best way to ensure a high degree of validity in the results because of the requirement for random assignment of participants and manipulation of the independent variable. There must be at least two groups in an experimental study, with one group serving as the control group (Gliner et al., 2009). Although there is a need to increase this type of research in education, it is difficult to employ random assignment in higher education. Additionally, there is a high degree of control required in an experimental study, which may not account for the contextual factors that affect a non-controlled educational environment.

Qualitative Designs

To understand phenomena that have little evidence in the literature, or to explore the multiple realities of the participants in DE, a qualitative approach may be chosen to answer the research question. The qualitative methodology chosen will vary based on the purpose of the research and may include description, phenomenology, grounded theory, narrative, or ethnography. Unlike quantitative research, an atheoretical approach is generally chosen for qualitative research so as to not bias the research findings. The contribution to theoretical advancement occurs after the completion of the study when the findings are related back to what is known in the literature. In DE, a qualitative approach may be used to understand student perspectives about aspects of DE such as interactions within the class. *Content analysis* has also been used to study discussion boards in DE for the level of student engagement, faculty engagement, and reflection.

Example of a Qualitative Study

Foronda and Lippincott (2014) used a qualitative narrative approach to explore the experience of nurse education certificate students who used the collaborate platform for interactive, synchronous videoconferencing within online courses. Forty-three students participated in one of four focus groups for data collection. The themes that emerged from the data regarding participant experiences of the videoconferencing were enjoyment, flexibility/convenience, interaction, a comparable or better than face-to-face experience, and technological problems.

Meta-Analysis/Metasynthesis

As the body of research grows in DE, researchers have begun to look critically at the methodology and findings of the studies that have been reported in the literature. In a *meta-analysis,* the results of individual studies are combined, and statistical analysis is done to generate findings from this combined set of data. Shachar (2008) stated that "[e]ducational measurement in general would benefit greatly, should researchers adopt: (1) [t]he practical usage of comparative effects sizes in their studies, in general, and (2) [t]he synthesizing of these effect sizes by means of a meta-analysis, in particular" (p. 4).

A *metasynthesis* pulls together findings from qualitative studies in common areas to understand phenomena. "Bringing together qualitative studies in a related area enables the nuances, taken-for-granted assumptions, and textured milieu of varying accounts to be exposed, described and explained in ways that bring fresh insights" (Walsh & Downe, 2005, p. 205).

Examples of Meta-Analysis and Metasynthesis

Shachar and Neumann (2010) completed a meta-analysis of the effect of blended learning on student outcomes in higher education. The sample included 96 studies published since 1990 with $k = 117$ effect sizes ($N = 10,800$ students). They found that the effect of blended learning on student achievement was low "but statistically greater than zero" (Shachar & Neumann, 2010, p. 115). They acknowledged that there were many confounding variables in the individual studies that could not be controlled for, which may have influenced the results.

Exploring the online teaching experience, De Gagne and Walters (2009) published a metasynthesis of studies between 2003 and 2008. They used the theory of critical thinking and community inquiry to frame their study. The sample included nine studies, four of which were published and five that were unpublished. The themes that emerged were work intensity, role changes, teaching strategies, and professional development.

MEASUREMENT

The strength of a study is directly related to the methods by which the variables in the research question are being measured. Investigators must select instruments that capture the dimensions of the variable as defined by either the theoretical framework guiding the study or as operationalized by the investigator in the research question. Although instruments exist that may be valid and reliable for traditional learning environments, their validity and reliability for the DE environment may need to be examined and empirically tested. New instruments that capture the unique aspects of the DE environment need to continue to be developed. For example, Ward-Smith, Schmer, Peterson, and Hart (2013) developed the Persistence Scale for Online Education (PSOE) (Cronbach's alpha = .729) to identify student ability to complete an online course.

Learning analytics have also shown promise in empirical studies in DE. "Learning analytics is the measurement, collection, analysis, and reporting of data about learners and their contexts, for purposes of understanding and optimizing learning and the environments in which it occurs" (Long & Siemens, 2011, p. 32). Data are obtained from learning management systems (LMS) and other sources to support decision making at the institutional level and understand student factors associated with success or risk. Student interactions in the LMS regarding student interactions in a course may be collected and potentially used to study engagement. These data may also be used to examine predictive factors related to student persistence in a DE class. Learning analytics collected over time has the opportunity to create Big Data sets, which may be available for investigators to use for modeling and other research studies.

FUTURE AREAS OF RESEARCH

Opportunities to advance the science of nursing education research in the area of nursing education can be framed using the I-E-O model of assessment of Astin. The model takes student inputs and the learning environment into consideration in the assessment of both cognitive and affective outcomes. Research about student outcomes is essential for the development of evidence-based strategies; however, it is no longer enough to just examine whether student learning outcomes or satisfaction with DE is as good as or better than traditional face-to-face learning experiences. Examining *why* DE is effective requires consideration of student and faculty characteristics, interaction, the design of the learning environment and/or educational intervention, and their relationship with student outcomes.

Inputs

Inputs are the learners' characteristics that are brought with them to the DE environment. Some of the variables studied are computer competency, motivation, self-directed or self-related learning, and learning style. However, descriptive information about these characteristics is not enough. It is important to study how these characteristics may influence engagement in the learning environment, as well as the achievement of student learning outcomes.

Environment

The experiences of the learners in distance learning are reflected in the environment of the I-E-O model of Astin. Engagement and interaction have been examined in DE research, both teacher-student and student-student. Although descriptive research in this area has been widely published, there is less evidence regarding the effect of engagement and interaction on student outcomes. It is also important to understand what this interaction looks like. What are the design elements of the course that motivated students to interact? Can those design elements be replicated and tested with a different group of learners with different characteristics? Could the outcomes of two courses with different design elements be compared? A massive open online course (MOOC) is one type of course design that has been studied in relation to student outcomes such as persistence. The "massive open online course (MOOC) is a model for delivering learning content online to any person who wants to take a course, with no limit on attendance" (Educause, n.d). The effectiveness of this type of course design warrants further study, particularly related to student outcomes. The environment also includes the technology used for course delivery, including the LMS. Student perceptions, engagement, and outcomes should be explored as new technologies are introduced.

Outputs

Outputs in Astin's I-E-O model can be categorized as either cognitive or affective. Cognitive outcomes are those that are related to knowledge acquisition or skill development and are usually measured using direct assessment. Performance on a test or the demonstration of a skill may be used to assess cognitive outcomes. Affective outcomes are those reflecting student perceptions and attitudes and may be measured using indirect measures such as opinion surveys, self-evaluation tools, and instruments designed to measure affective outcomes like attitudes and confidence. Russell (2015) stated the following: "Future research in online nursing education needs to expand outcomes evaluation away from the affective learning domain. The established research in this area has demonstrated positive affective learning outcomes, but much of it is perceived learning versus actual learning" (p. 19). Not only is it important to focus on cognitive outcomes, but investigators must also look for the connection of those outcomes to the design of the course and the characteristics of the learners.

CONCLUSIONS AND IMPLICATIONS

As technologies and broadband improve, the trend for an increase in the use of DE is expected to continue. DE allows nursing education to reach rural and medically underserved areas, preparing practitioners to practice at higher levels while meeting the health care needs of the underserved areas. Many students are also choosing DE to meet the flexibility of their lifestyles. It is clear that DE is here to stay. To continue to improve learning in DE, it is imperative that nurse investigators continue to find evidence for the best practices for teaching and learning at a distance. The need to use a common language in conducting and disseminating these studies is clear—so that future researchers can build on the evidence and for inclusion in multisite studies or meta-analyses. Improving the rigor of designs, measurement, and use of theoretical frameworks to guide the research is also essential. Through carefully designed studies, the state of the science of DE in nursing can be advanced.

References

Allen, I. E., & Seaman, J. (2015). *Grade level: Tracking online education in the United States*. Retrieved June 10, 2016, from http://www.onlinelearningsurvey.com/reports/gradelevel.pdf

American Association of Colleges of Nursing. (2007). *Alliance for nursing accreditation statement on distance education policies*. Retrieved June 10, 2016, from http://www.aacn.nche.edu/education-resources/distance-education-policies

Armstrong, M., Gessner, B., & Cooper, S. (2000). POTS, PANS, and PEARLS: The nursing profession's rich history with distance education for a new century of nursing. *Journal of Continuing Education in Nursing, 31*(2), 63–70.

Bernard, R., Abrami, P., Lou, Y, Borokhovski, E., Wade, A., Wozney, L., et al. (2004). How does distance education compare with classroom instruction? A meta-analysis of the empirical literature. *Review of Educational Research, 74*, 379–439. doi:10.3102/00346543074003379

Bozkurt, A., Akgun-Ozbek, E., Yilmazel, S., Erdogdu, E., Ucar, H., Guler, E., et al. (2015). Trends in distance education research: A content analysis of journals 2009–2013. *International Review of Research in Open and Distributed Learning, 16*, 330–363.

Broome, M., Ironside, P., & McNelis, A. (2012). Research in nursing education: State of the Science. *Journal of Nursing Education, 51*, 521–524. doi:10.3928/01484834-20120820-10

Cameron, N. (2013). Comparative descriptors of applicants and graduates of online and face-to-face master of science in nursing programs. *Nursing Education Perspectives, 84*, 372–376. doi:10.5480/11-518.1

De Gagne, J., & Walters, K. (2009). Online teaching experience: A qualitative metasynthesis (QMS). *Journal of Online Teaching and Learning, 5*, 577–589. Available at http://jolt.merlot.org/vol5no4/degagne_1209.pdf

Educause. (n.d.). *Massive open online course (MOOC)*. Retrieved June 10, 2016, from https://library.educause.edu/topics/teaching-and-learning/massive-open-online-course-mooc

Foronda, C., & Lippincott, C. (2014). Graduate nursing students' experience with synchronous interactive videoconferencing within online courses. *Quarterly Review of Distance Education, 15*(2), 1–8.

Gliner, J., Morgan, G., & Leech, N. (2009). Research methods in applied settings: An integrated approach to design and analysis (2nd ed.). New York: Routledge.

Grove, S., Burns, N., & Gray, J. (2012). *The practice of nursing research: Appraisal, synthesis, and generation of evidence* (7th ed.). Atlanta, GA: Elsevier.

Hunter, J., & Krantz, S. (2010). Constructivism in cultural competence education. *Journal of Nursing Education, 49*, 207–214. doi:10.3928/01484834-20100115-06

Johnson, B. (2000). *It's (beyond) time to drop the terms causal-comparative and correlational research in education*. Retrieved June 10, 2016, from http://itforum.coe.uga.edu/paper43/paper43.html

Long, P. D., & Siemens, G. (2011). Penetrating the fog: Analytics in learning and education.

Educause Review. Retrieved June 10, 2016, from http://www.educause.edu/ero/article/penetrating-fog-analytics-learning-and-education

Mayadas, F., Miller, G., & Sener, J. (2015). Definitions of e-learning courses and programs version 2.0 April 4, 2015, developed for discussion within the online learning community. *Online Learning Consortium*. Retrieved June 10, 2016, from http://onlinelearningconsortium.org/updated-e-learning-definitions-2/#

Means, B., Toyama, Y., Murphy, R., & Baki, M. (2013). The effectiveness of online and blended learning: A meta-analysis of the empirical literature. *Teachers College Record, 115*, 1–47.

National League for Nursing. (2016). *NLN research priorities in nursing education*, 2016–2019. Retrieved June 10, 2016, from http://www.nln.org/docs/default-source/professional-development-programs/nln-research-priorities-in-nursing-education-single-pages.pdf?sfvrsn=2

Patterson, B., & Krouse, A. (2012). Student outcomes of distance learning in nursing education. *CIN: Computers,Informatics, Nursing, 30*, 475–488. doi:10.1097/NXN.0b013e3182573ad4

Poulin, R. (2015). Highlights of distance education enrollment trends from IPEDS fall 14. *WCET*. Retrieved June 10, 2016, from https://wcetblog.wordpress.com/2015/12/21/ipeds-fall-2014-de-highlights

Russell, B. (2015). The who, what, and how of evaluation within online nursing education: State of the science. *Journal of Nursing Education, 54*, 13–21. doi:10.3928/01484834-20141228-02

Shachar, M. (2008). Meta-analysis: The preferred method of choice for the assessment of distance learning quality factors. *International Review of Research in Open and Distance Learning, 9*(3), 1–15. Available at http://www.irrodl.org/index.php/irrodl/article/view/493/1147

Shachar, M., & Neumann, Y. (2010). Twenty years of research on the academic performance differences between traditional and distance learning: Summative meta-analysis and trend examination. *Journal of Online Teaching and Learning, 6*, 318–334. Available at http://jolt.merlot.org/vol6no2/shachar_0610.pdf

Shadish, W., Cook, T., & Campbell, D. (2002). *Experimental and quasi-experimental designs for generalized causal inference.* Boston: Houghton Mifflin.

Sitzmann, T., Kraiger, K., Stewart, D., & Wisher, R. (2006). The comparative effectiveness of web-based and classroom instruction: A meta-analysis. *Personnel Psychology, 59*, 623–664. doi:10.1111/j.1744-6570.2006.00049.x

Thurmond, V. (2002). Considering theory in assessing quality of web-based courses. *Nurse Educator, 27*(1), 20–24.

U.S. Department of Education. (2009). *Evaluation of evidence-based practices in online learning: A meta-analysis and review of online learning studies.* Washington, DC: Author. Available at https://www2.ed.gov/rschstat/eval/tech/evidence-based-practices/finalreport.pdf

Walsh, D., & Downe, S. (2005). Meta-synthesis method for qualitative research: A literature review. *Journal of Advanced Nursing, 50*, 204–211. doi:10.1111/j.1365-2648.2005.03380.x

Ward-Smith, P., Schmer, C., Peterson, J., & Hart, C. (2013). Persistence among graduate nursing students enrolled in an online course. *Journal of Nursing Education and Practice, 3*, 48–52. doi:10.5430/jnep.v3n9p48

Wells, M., & Dellinger, A. (2011). The effect of type of learning environment on perceived learning among graduate nursing students. *Nursing Education Perspectives, 32*, 406–410. doi:10.5480/1536-5026-32.6.406

Yucha, C., Schneider, B., Smyer, T., Kowalski, S., & Stowers, E. (2011). Methodological quality and scientific impact of quantitative nursing education research over 18 months. *Nursing Education Perspectives, 32*, 362–368. doi:10.5480/1536-5026-32.6.362

Zhao, Y., Lei, J., Yan, B., Lai, C., & Tan, H. (2005). What makes the difference? A practical analysis of research on the effectiveness of distance education. *Teachers College Record, 107*, 1836–1884. doi:10.1111/j.1467-9620.2005.00544.x